The 90 day No Equipment workout plan For Women

G.M Zollo

Table of Contents

Introduction

The first thing I want to make 100% clear is that no matter who you are, no matter how long you have battled with your weight, and no matter how many times you have failed at changing your body to a level that you're happy with, no matter how "slow" you think your metabolism is, you CAN lose fat, get toned and completely change the shape of your body.

Many people fail in this space because of two reasons: they are taking the wrong advice and implementing the wrong strategies, and the second, those who are following the correct methods, aren't giving enough time. Crash diets, mixed with the wrong type of training and supplement, promise the world or quick and easy weight loss, but deliver an atlas of health problems. This is a combination that is promoted heavily by the marketing teams of mainstream fitness programs and supplement companies. Unfortunately, they continue to fool many people over and over again.

Building your perfect body with toned legs, a nicely shaped butt, and toned arms at its core, is such a simple process. It has been made out to be complicated to keep the fitness industry's economy running for many years to come. They thrive on your failure so that they can prey on your emotional state with their next supplement or their next overpriced workout machine advertised on the late-night shopping channel. The facts are that losing body fat, increasing muscle tone, and improving your health are the same now as what it was 100 years ago and will be the same in 100 years. The human body and its mechanics don't change, but unfortunately, good marketing in the wrong hands leads you down the path of failure before you even begin your journey.

Throughout this book, I will go through what the "experts" preach has to be done to transform your body and why that's wrong. I will show you why these methods make it harder to stick to your diet and workout program and why in many cases, they actually lead you to eat more than you normally would, taking you further away from your goal.

You will discover two different ways to tackle your nutrition. The first is fail-proof but does require a little more planning. It is for those people like myself who like to geek out on numbers and are happy to take a little more time with the finer details in their weight loss program. This is the method I used for my transformation, where I was able to lose over 50 lbs. in 8 months. This guarantees success. Follow it, and you are certain to lose weight.

The second option isn't as time-consuming and is still very effective, although you will have to be a bit more mindful of what and how you're eating, along with your energy levels and mood throughout the day. I normally recommend this once someone enters the maintenance phase of their transformation, but it can also easily be adapted to the transformation phase.

Once we have your nutrition out of the way, we will look at the actual workout. This program is specifically designed so that you don't require any equipment whatsoever, and it can be followed anywhere at any time, regardless of your financial situation or the lack of equipment at your disposal. I have designed it to take you from a complete beginner all the way up to a warrior with strength that will stand the test of time and have you able to tackle any physical demand life throws at you with confidence. It will increase your longevity and slow down the aging process. Along with that all-important functional strength, you will also gain the bi-product, which is that you're going to look pretty damn good as well.

The great thing is that it's all done with a minimalist approach, so you won't need to spend hours and hours per week exercising. Those long grueling workouts 6 days a week are not necessary or sustainable, so why do it? Living a healthy lifestyle should enhance your life and make it better, not take away from it by getting in the way and preventing you from enjoying life. I don't want you stressing about getting your workout every day or if a particular food is going to make you gain fat, and I have structured this program accordingly.

Throughout this book, I will teach you how to completely transform your figure and completely change and improve the quality of your life. The program is based on being lean and strong, as I believe strength is the key to longevity. It's one of the first things to deteriorate as we get older, so getting on top of that and maintaining it is the key to staying younger and being active and pain-free for longer.

Your journey will culminate in a fit, strong, athletic mother, daughter, aunt, or sister looking back at you in the mirror. It will be a totally new you, no gyms, no equipment, no fuss, no excuses, and certainly no magic pills. Your body weight, 3 days a week, and a consistent effort and commitment to yourself are the only things required.

Let's do this.

Facebook Group

The best way to succeed at anything is to surround yourself with people on the same path. That's why I have created a private Facebook group for people serious about transforming their bodies and changing their lifestyles for the better.

This will be an opportunity to communicate with myself as well as other people aiming to rebuild their bodies from the ground up. This group will be an important tool for you when it comes to getting over any hurdles and challenges you hit along the way. I will do my absolute best to keep you on track. I will answer any questions you have as well as help you with any exercise replacements if there is a part of the program you are unable to do due to injury or your current strength level. Your success is my success, and I want this for you.

Just click here or scan the QR code below, and it will take you straight to my group. From there, you answer 3 very simple questions, so I know you're serious about this, and I will accept you into the group.

Free 28 Day Habit Tracker and 30% off My One-on-One Coaching Program

The average time between people taking on a body transformation program and giving up is around 3 weeks. This is due to the learning curve that comes at the start, mainly with working out your nutritional numbers and knowing what to eat. When people don't get the quick result, they are after initially, their motivation dies, and eventually, they quit.

I want you to build momentum from the very start, so I have put together a 28-day habit tracker designed to help you bust through all of the noise in the fitness industry and prevent overwhelm. This will give you the 5 must-do's that you need to focus on daily to get in shape, and ticking off as many of these boxes as u can each day ensures that they become a natural part of your life by the end of those 28 days. When you pair this with the minimalist style of the program I have outlined in this book, you are guaranteed to get results without fitness taking over your life.

On top of this, I will also send you my 21-Day Fat Loss Kickstart Plan to give you a head start with your nutrition while you go through the workout, as well as my Fix Your Nutrition eBook. This eBook goes more in-depth into all areas of nutrition and supplementation.

As a special thank you for purchasing this book, I would also like to offer you a 30% discount on my one-on-one coaching program.

Click here or scan the QR code below to get your discount code and download your other goodies.

If you have problems downloading it, email me at Michael.zollo@hotmail.com, and I will get it to you ASAP.

Chapter 1:

Why Workout?

Working out isn't just about losing weight and toning up. It's about improving and maintaining your overall mental, emotional, and physical well-being.

Women that work out regularly get some amazing rewards. If you're new to exercising on a regular basis, some of these might surprise you: improving your skin, sleep quality, and mental health is just the start.

There are plenty of reasons why you should be incorporating exercise into your daily or weekly routine. Here are a few:

Your Skin

Everyone loves that feeling you get straight after a good workout, your endorphins are released, and you get a great post-work glow in your skin. Regular exercise can do amazing things for your skin.

This is because working out gets your heart pumping and increases circulation, giving your skin a good hit of oxygenated blood. Upping your blood flow helps to nourish your skin cells as your blood carries oxygen and nutrients to cells throughout your body, including your skin. This is one of the many reasons exercises makes you look and feel vibrant, both inside and out.

Another way working out can help your skin is sweat. Sweat helps your pores flush out oil, dirt, and bacteria that can lead to spots or blemishes. Make sure you have a good scrub after exercising to wash away all the bad stuff you sweat out.

Improves Mental Health

Exercise is known to have an extremely positive affect for those suffering from mental health issues. It can help with things such as boosting mental clarity to relieving stress.

When you work out, neurotransmitters called endorphins are released that help change a person's mood positively. The amounts released vary with the type of exercise and intensity of your workout. There have been a few studies in this space with conflicting outcomes. Some studies have found that those who do an hour of HIIT training (high intensity interval training) experienced a significant increase in endorphin release compared with those who completed an hour of less demanding exercise. Although there have also been some studies that have found that it may not be the higher endorphin levels that make you feel good after your workout. It's been suggested that even though endorphin levels are higher after physical activity, they can't pass through the blood-brain barrier. Either way, exercise also releases a chemical cocktail of dopamine, norepinephrine, and serotonin, which all help with mood regulation.

As for stress and anxiety, something that I deal with personally, exercise is a tried and tested way to break the cycle of stress and worry. It helps you to relax your muscles, relieve tension, and enjoy a mental break from the negative thoughts of stress and anxiety.

Better Sleep

According to The National Sleep Foundation, exercise works great for improving the quality of your sleep. As well as tiring you out so your body wants sleep to recover, your body temperature is raised a few degrees during exercise. When your body temperature drops back down later in the day, this can trigger feelings of sleepiness and helps you doze off easily.

Why is getting good quality sleep so important? The body repairs itself while you sleep. A night of good sleep can enhance your memory and decrease bodily inflammation. Most human growth hormone (HGH) is released when you sleep, a hormone that plays a key role in growth, body composition, cell repair, metabolism, and more. On top of that, these hormones are what keep our skin and muscles young. It's also been shown that a lack of sleep consistently can increase the chances of things like dementia and Alzheimer's.

Beat the Cramps

Many women decide to skip their workout during that time of the month, but actually, it's completely ok to exercise during your period, and it could even provide some benefits.

You may find that you can exercise at a higher intensity during your period than at other times of the month, partly due to changes in hormone levels. Getting a good dose of mood-boosting hormones is just the start. Some studies show that many women have reported fewer painful cramps during their period if they exercise regularly.

That being said, staying in tune with your body is important so you notice any obvious changes. Exercising too much or too intensely can cause you to miss your period or stop your period altogether. This is more common in professional athletes and those who do many hours of intense training per week. This doesn't normally apply to the average person looking to lose a few pounds and improve their health unless it's mixed with extreme crash dieting.

Chapter 2:

Bodyweight Training vs Weight Training

Over the years, as gyms have become increasingly popular, bodyweight training seems to have been given this stigma around it that it's not as effective when building lean muscle and creating a toned athletic body.

This is wrong; bodyweight training is unbelievably effective when it comes to transforming your body. It's the purest form of strength, and if you know how to do it correctly, you don't need 90% of the machines you see in the gym.

Understand this; resistance is resistance. If you do a set of heavy barbell squats or a barbell press, your body doesn't know how much weight you have added to the bar; all it knows is that there is tension there, it is hard, and it is going to require a certain amount of effort to complete the movement. The same goes with a bodyweight exercise; your body doesn't know if you're doing a standard bodyweight push-up or a bench press. All it knows is if it's intense and challenging, it doesn't change the signals sent to your body.

One of the big benefits of bodyweight training is that it reduces the risk of injury. It's great for keeping your joints and ligaments healthy long-term compared to focusing on weight training. Bodyweight training helps keep your body in proper proportion and ensures you have a solid foundation with your core strength that you can build on safely.

On top of this, bodyweight training recruits more muscle fibers to perform a movement than its weight training counterpart. This is due to it being a closed-chain exercise. This means that your body is moving through space rather than a barbell or dumbbell. An example of this is when you do a push-up, your body moves up and down while your hands are in a fixed position on the floor. Now compare that to a bench press, which is the same movement with the same muscles being worked, but in this case, it is your body that's in a fixed position on a bench, and it's the barbell and your hands that are moving through space. Not only does this make the bodyweight version great for building lean muscle, but it leaves fewer margins for error with your form and, as a result, makes it a safer alternative.

Another great part of bodyweight training is that you can do it anywhere. If you travel a lot for work, you can keep your training on track in your hotel room; if it's a nice day outside, you can train at the park or the beach and catch some vitamin D instead of being inside the 4 walls of the gym. If you're someone that does enjoy weight training, then bodyweight training can be worked into your program as well to create an effective hybrid program. It's also a great replacement if you're busy and can't make it to the gym for a few days; you can easily fit in a quick 15-20 minute intense bodyweight workout at home and get great strength and conditioning benefits as well as giving your body a different stimulus to your normal training.

Bodyweight training is unmatched when it comes to building coordination, athleticism, and core strength. To manipulate your body through certain movements, you build your athletic base, and your core has no choice but to get stronger along with it. This translates into a higher level of performance with the way your body moves in everyday life.

Am I saying weight training is no good? Not, weight training is great and has many benefits; I still do it myself throughout the week. It has its place, but it is a luxury. True strength is built upon being able to master your body weight and being able to throw it around like it's nothing.

The Problem With Most Bodyweight Programs

There are plenty of bodyweight programs out there, but the truth is that most miss the mark completely. The two ways they are normally set out are in training for high reps or in a circuit HIIT format where its main goal is to smash you as hard as possible to burn the maximum amount of calories in each workout.

As you get stronger at a particular exercise, these programs focus on building up more reps to increase intensity and challenge you. This is fine to a certain extent, but when training to increase lean muscle mass, which is what people often mean when they say they want to be toned, doing anything more than 12-15 reps on an exercise becomes pointless. It changes the intention of the workout.

Once you get past 15 reps, you avoid building lean muscle and strength and focus more on conditioning and muscle endurance. That's fine if that's your goal, but I'm tipping that you here because you want to improve the aesthetics of your body and build strength that will help ensure you are turning back the clock as you get older. If you can build up to 30,40, or 50 pushups, the first 70% of that set is probably really easy, and you only recruit the maximum amount of muscle fibers in the last few reps. Pointless if your goal is to build serious strength and change your body composition.

The second way that bodyweight programs are set out is in either a circuit or HIIT style. This takes you even further away from your goal if you want to be strong and athletic. These programs are cardio-based and will increase your strength initially, but nothing too far behind that since you constantly move from one exercise to another with little to no rest in between sets to recover. Circuits and HIIT training have their place. If your goal is to get as fit as possible but lose fat and build muscle, they will not get It done. In the next chapter, I will explore why cardio routines should not be your focus if losing weight is your goal.

Moving on to the next issue with many bodyweight programs, which show up more in the circuit-style setups, is that they are filled with 30 to 50 exercises. The main reason is to create variation and stop people from getting bored. The thing with the fitness industry is that people feel like they need to keep recreating the wheel by creating new workout formats and exercises for different body parts to keep the fitness industry going. The basics are all you need; they worked 100 yrs. ago and will work 100 years from now.

To build a great body, you only need a few basic compound movements that bring multiple muscle groups into it and allow the whole body to be worked. The trick is to change each movement to a more challenging variation once you reach a certain level rather than just endlessly increasing reps.

No doubt, when you see the workout later, you're probably going to think it's too basic but remember, it doesn't mean easy, and the lack of variety of 50 different exercises means you're going to get good at the moves that matter when it comes to body composition and performance with everyday tasks.

Chapter 3:

Busting the Myths

In this chapter, I would like to look at some of the myths plaguing the fitness industry and overcomplicating the whole process.

Cardio is Best for Weight Loss

This is a big one, walk into any gym, and the battle lines are drawn. Cardio or strength training? Which is the most important in changing your body? For many years and still, to this day, cardio is looked at as number one when it comes to losing weight, while strength training is seen purely for bodybuilders looking to get big. WRONG.

People think this is because you burn more calories in a cardio workout than in a traditional strength session; your heart rate remains higher for a longer period. Although this is true, what people forget to look at is the afterburn or the flow-on effect of a workout. A good strength training session will have you burn calories faster throughout the day, well beyond your workout session. After a cardio workout, the rate at which you burn calories will slow down to your normal rate within 20 minutes of finishing your workout.

On top of this, a transformation built purely on cardio training alone will result in what's referred to in the industry as a "skinny fat" body. This means you will simply become a smaller version of what you were before beginning your weight loss journey. Although you will lose scale weight, it will come from a mixture of lean muscle and fat, meaning the shape of your body won't change; you won't build toned arms and legs or have a tight waist. Those results come from strength training and, of course, diet.

Strength training with barbells, dumbbells, pin-loaded machines, or your body weight is king for all aspects of changing your body aesthetically. Walking is the only cardio necessary which I will go into a little later.

Doing too much cardio, such as running on the treadmill, also makes it harder to stick to your diet because doing large amounts of cardio increases plasma ghrelin. This is known as the hunger hormone, and when its levels are raised, your hunger increases, making it harder to eat at the calorie deficit required to lose weight.

If you want to focus on fitness levels simultaneously, there is another option you can get the best of both worlds and structure your workouts to have both a strength and cardio aspect to them. You can do this by performing a super set where you group multiple strength exercises without a break and then have your break at the end. The key here is to not group too many; otherwise, it leans towards being similar to a circuit I explained earlier; I would keep it to two exercises only.

Meal Timing and Eating Small Meals Regularly Matters

This one has only recently been debunked, but for many years, we were told that to lose weight, you must eat 6 small meals daily every 3 hours.

The logic behind this was that your body uses energy to digest food, so putting food in your body every 3 hours means you will be regularly using energy (calories) to break down those foods and, in turn, burning more calories throughout the day.

It was also said that having large amounts of time between those meals, your body would go into starvation mode. This is because it doesn't know when the next meal is coming in, so your metabolism will adjust by slowing down to ensure you always have energy when needed.

The whole starvation mode concept is real, but we now know that it kicks in from eating too few calories overall throughout the entire day and has nothing to do with how or when you consume those calories. This is why when people go on some of these fad crash diets and eat next to nothing trying to lose weight, they generally get results for about a week or two, and then it completely stops soon after. Since meal timing no longer plays a part in losing weight, intermittent fasting has become a popular choice when choosing a lifestyle that is not only sustainable but healthy at the same time. I follow this method and have had great success with it. It's not for everyone, though, and I would ask you to do your research if you think it's something you want to try. There are plenty of free articles online, and I also have a couple of books on the topic if you are interested in learning more. I will leave the link to my 16/8 book, the most common form of intermittent fasting.

Intermittent fasting 16/8

If You Eat Healthy You Can Eat as Much as You Want

This myth causes heartache, with many people struggling to lose weight. The number of times I have had people tell me that they only eat healthy, clean foods, yet they haven't lost any weight or, even worse, are putting on weight. They cut out sugar, desserts, soda, deep-fried foods, etc., and they still can't lose weight. On top of that, they are miserable with what they eat, making it harder to stick with anyway.

You will get different opinions on this, no doubt, but at the end of the day, in the calorie world (not the health world), the calories in a gram of carbohydrate, protein, and fat are the same no matter where it comes from, be it a healthy serving of quinoa or from a sugary chocolate chip cookie.

Those calories add up to your total caloric intake, and if that number is more than what you have burned off that day, then you won't lose weight no matter how "healthy" you have eaten.

Important note Even though the above implies you don't have to eat clean 100% of the time, your diet should still be made up of mostly healthy, clean foods. This will not only boost your energy levels and support good heart health, but it adds volume to your foods, giving you the most bang for your buck with calories. Healthy, clean foods tend to keep you fuller for longer and minimize the chance of a mid-afternoon binge session that will undo all of your previous good work. If you can stick to the 80/20 rule regarding healthy, clean foods compared to guilty pleasures, then you should be well on your way to success.

Women Get Bulky Lifting Weights

This is probably the most frustrating myth out of all of them for most personal trainers. Whenever I get a new female client, and I add an appropriate amount of strength training into their program, I often get that concerned look staring back at me, followed by them reinforcing the fact that they want to lose weight and don't want to get bulky or have big arms.

The facts are that women don't have the testosterone that men do, meaning strength training will not have the same outcome. For a female to get bulky and overly muscular, it will require a number of things, the first being years and years of living, breathing, and bleeding a bodybuilding or powerlifting lifestyle, and the second is a diet that matches that insane level of dedication where they eat at a caloric surplus (the exact opposite to what you would do when trying to lose weight) and three, more than likely a course of steroids to compliment the previous two points.

Strength training will give the everyday female a nicely toned and fit-looking body with a metabolism that will allow you to not have to stress over every little mouthful of food that enters your body to maintain it - Take home message - do not skip training.

Crunches and Other Ab Exercises Reduces Belly Fat

You need to train your abs to lose the fat around your abs. Once again, a popular and common theory but a very incorrect one'd

Specific ab exercises, whether crunches or a high-tech rip-off gadget on late-night TV, will strengthen and tone your abs. However, you will not be able to see that tone while you have a high level of body fat covering them, and those abs machines and extra sit-ups have no more influence on reducing body fat around your stomach than pushups, squats, or jumping jacks have.

Don't be fooled by the fact that those ab machines you see are being marketed by some fitness model who somehow manages to maintain that big glowing smile while using it. The body they present to you in these infomercials is not a result of using that machine. It results from working the entire body consistently and having a low body fat percentage from a targeted diet.

While we are at it, this goes for any other body part as well; you cannot spot reduction on a specific body part, your body will choose where and when the weight comes off, and unfortunately, the places we carry the most weight and are most self-conscious about can often be the last place it comes off. It's frustrating, I know, but it is what it is; just understand that eventually it will happen, so stay consistent

You Can't Eat Carbs at Night

The thought process behind this is that carbohydrates are a source of energy, and if you eat them at night, then you're less likely to burn them off as you are less active at night, resulting in them being stored as body fat. The timing of your food intake will not do anything to prevent weight loss. Your meals should be high in protein with a good balance of clean carbohydrate sources and healthy fats and veggies to complement that; if you enjoy eating them at night, then go for it; I do.

The More Exercise the Better

This myth doesn't only plague the fitness industry but also many other areas of life, the whole "more is better" concept. When it comes to changing the shape of your body, too much exercise can make it harder and hinder your results. High-intensity workouts 6-7 days per week mixed with a large calorie deficit will damage your hormones and ensure you hit a brick wall with your progress sooner rather than later.

We recover, repair, and get stronger when we rest, and if you're training 6 days per week, you're eating into your recovery time. This will lead to many of the negative side effects mentioned earlier in this chapter and injuries that will only set you back further. This becomes an even more valid point as we get older.

On top of how many workouts you do per week, you should look at how long each of those sessions goes for and the intensity. I have often seen people in the gym for 2-3 hours; there is no need to go past 45-60 minutes of intense exercise at a time (not including a light warm-up or stretching). When you go beyond that, your body can start to feed off its muscle tissue for energy which is not what you want. This defeats the purpose, as we are trying to use our stored fat for energy while maintaining and building lean muscle. If you enjoy exercising like I do and want to train daily, you certainly can; it just takes a more conscious approach to your workouts. Some sessions will have to be more of a recovery session at a much lower intensity level to ensure you're still able to recover; this program works on a 3 session per week schedule, so overtraining will not occur.

Why is it So Hard to Drop Fat?

Now that we have covered some of the myths about what creates fat loss and how simple the process is, you might ask yourself, "since the process is so basic, why is it so hard to achieve and sustain"?

Being in a calorie deficit is done through taking control of your diet, you might have heard the saying "you can't out exercise a bad diet", this is 100% true, it means you might put in the work and have a great workout, burning 600 plus calories but those 600 calories can be undone pretty quickly with one meal if you're not mindful about what and how much you're eating

Unfortunately we live in a society where we are faced with an abundance of quick convenient low quality foods with very little nutritious value. These foods are usually small in volume but extremely high in calories, meaning a blow can happen quickly and without knowing it. Even worse, you won't feel satiated at the end of it, leading you to reach for more food of the same quality. Making things worse, getting a hold of these foods has never been easier, a simple swipe of a credit card and an Uber eats account will take care of that for you and you don't even need to leave your couch to do so.

If you don't take control of your diet habits, your chances of success are not good, but by being mindful of what, and how much you put in your body, then you will be in complete control and increase your chances of completely rebuilding your body from the ground up.

The free PDF I mentioned earlier in the book will give you the tools you need to understand food and make your nutrition work for you and your lifestyle rather than following some other generic cookie cutter 1200 calorie crash diet that many other workout books have. These will leave you low on energy, constantly starving and thinking about food all day long, we only have so much willpower to give so don't make that mistake.

Chapter 4:

How to Use This Book

This book is laid out in a progression that takes you from a pure beginner with very little strength to a lean and functionally strong woman with great muscle tone to go with it.

The 90-day program is all about building solid strength with pure bodyweight movements. Each exercise will have a progression of 3 to 4 movements that you can work through as you get stronger. You will see these progressions later in this book.

These exercises will be grouped to make an upper and lower-body workout. You will do 3 workouts total per week on alternate days. One week you will do the upper body twice and the lower body once before you swap it around the following week by doing the lower body twice and the upper body once.

As your strength increases in a particular exercise and you can reach the prescribed number of reps comfortably to the point where you can do 3 to 5 more with solid technique, you will go to the next more challenging progression of that exercise. You might find with some of the exercises that there is quite a big jump from one progression to the next; if this is the case, you can do a couple of things. First, stay on the progression you have been making and build up more reps beyond what I have prescribed, then move on to the more challenging progression further down the track. Alternatively, instead of adding more reps, you can add some external resistance, such as wearing a backpack filled with whatever you need to add weight and make that movement more challenging. If you are strong enough to do the next progression but fall short on the set rep range, I would get you to do whatever reps you can before finishing the rest of the set with the previous easier progression.

You must track your workouts, writing down how many reps you're hitting on each set of each exercise. You will soon see this won't be a linear process. Some movements are easier to progress in than others, and you might get stuck on a particular movement for a few weeks before breaking through it.

Don't rush it; make sure you're dominating a movement before moving up. If I have set 3 sets of 8 reps for a certain exercise, then make sure those 3 sets of 8 are strong with a good form where that last rep isn't a complete struggle to complete before moving up. As mentioned earlier, I would encourage you to reach a point where you could probably hit a few more reps before moving on.

Along with your strength sessions, you will want to aim for 8000 to 10,000 steps each day and do some stretching for recovery. If you have some type of smartwatch, then you can track your steps on that; if not, just try to go for a designated 45-60 min brisk walk 2-3 days per week on your off days and try to walk every opportunity you can each day to increase your step count? Walking is not an essential part of the program for transforming your body. Still, it is an essential part of your overall health, plus it will allow for extra fat burning, and being such a low-intensity form of cardio, it will not interfere with your recovery from your all-important strength workouts.

Remember, although it's a 90-day program, getting to the more advanced movements will probably take longer. You may not even be able to get to some of those movements, and that's ok. This is about becoming the leanest, strongest version of you that you can be and keeping that for life.

Now onto the routine, below is how you will schedule this throughout your week, and after that, I will have each exercise progression listed with a photo, description, and a clickable link so you can watch a video of the exercise being done.

Here is an example schedule

Week 1

Sunday	45-60 min walk
Monday	Upper Body Strength Workout
Tuesday	45-60 min walk
Wednesday	Lower Body Strength Workout
Thursday	Off
Friday	Upper Body Strength Workout
Saturday	45-60 min walk

Week 2

Sunday	45-60 min walk
Monday	Lower Body Strength Workout
Tuesday	45-60 min walk
Wednesday	Upper Body Strength Workout
Thursday	Off
Friday	Lower Body Strength Workout
Saturday	45-60 min walk

You can set out your plan in whatever way you need to make it work for you. The only rule I would say you need to follow is ensuring the strength workouts are done on alternate days.

Chapter 5:

The Exercises and Progressions

The Pushup Progression

The primary muscles worked here are your pectoral muscles (chest), and the secondary muscles worked are your anterior deltoid (front of shoulder) and your triceps (back of your upper arm)

Progression One – <u>Push Ups On Your Knees</u>

Instructions

Begin with your knees on the floor and your arms straight with your hands flat on the ground beneath your shoulders.

Engage your core and slowly lower your chest and stomach to the ground until your elbows are bent at approximately 90 degrees. Push back up to the starting position until your arms are straight.

Make sure your butt is in line with your stomach and chest at the bottom of the movement, do not leave your butt in the air.

Have your elbows positioned around 45 degrees so halfway between being in line with your shoulders and the side of your body; you mustn't have them flared out in line with your shoulders as it will place increased strain on your shoulder joints risking injury.

Repeat for the prescribed number of reps.

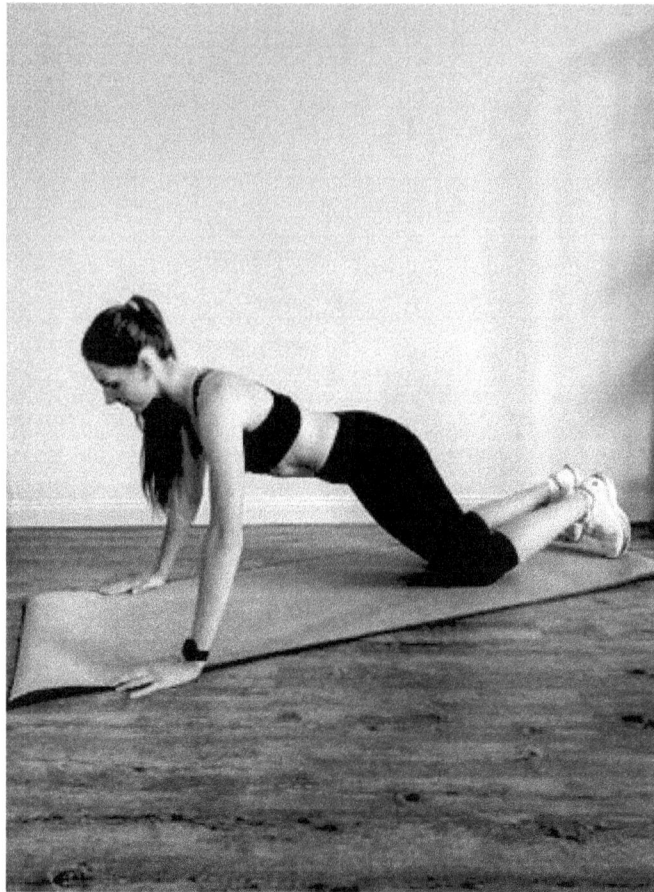

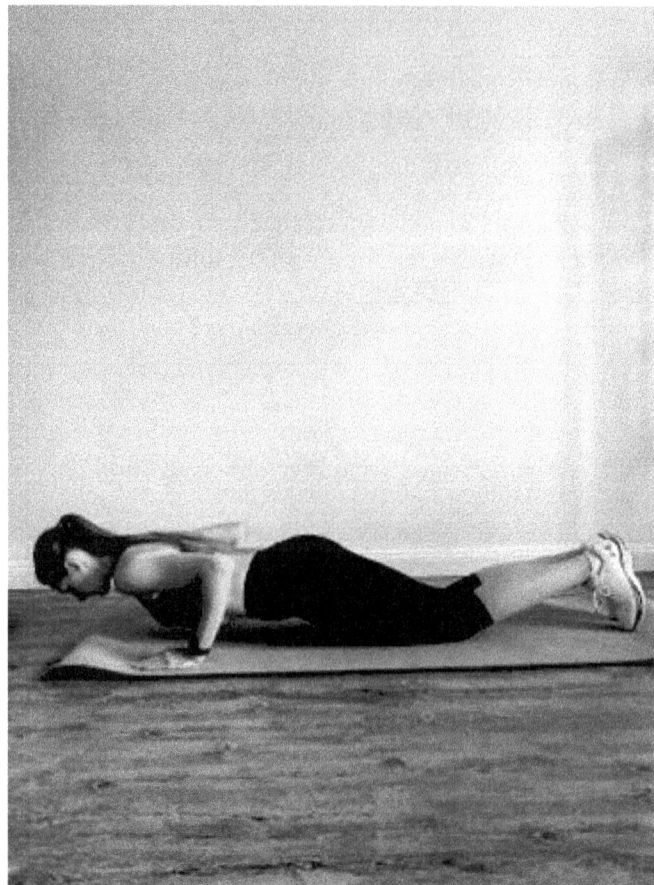

Progression Two – <u>Pushups On Your Toes</u>

Instructions

Begin by getting into a plank position with your arms and body straight and your hands flat on the ground beneath your shoulders. You will have your legs straight, balancing on your toes.

As with performing pushups on your knees, you will engage your core and lower your chest towards the ground until your elbows are bent approximately 90 degrees. The same caution must be taken with the positioning of your elbows, making sure they are not flared out in line with your shoulders, as many people do.

From here, push back up to the starting position with your arms straight, ensuring your lower back doesn't slouch or your butt isn't stuck in the air.

Repeat for the prescribed number of reps.

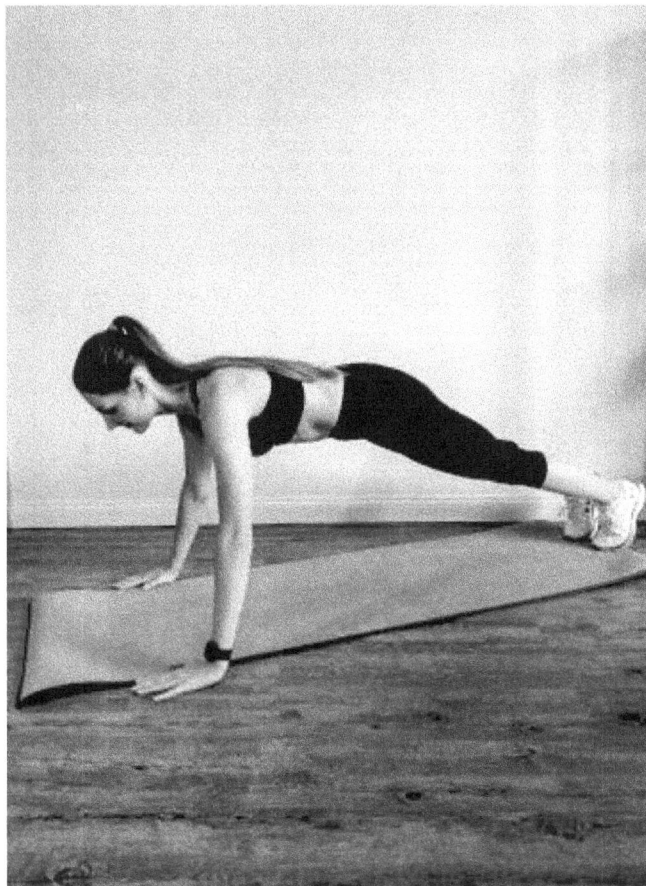

Progression Three – <u>Pushups With Your Feet Elevated.</u>

Instructions

Begin by getting into a plank position, with your body and arms straight and your hands flat on the ground beneath your shoulders. For this progression, you will have your legs straight and balancing on your toes with your feet elevated; either your couch, a step, or a chair is fine; the higher your feet are elevated, the more complex the movement becomes.

Start by engaging your core and lowering your down towards the ground until your chest is a few inches from the floor with your elbows at 45 degrees, around halfway between your shoulders and the sides of your body.

From here, push back up to the starting position with your arms straight, ensuring your lower back remains straight and doesn't slouch throughout the movement.

Repeat for the prescribed number of reps.

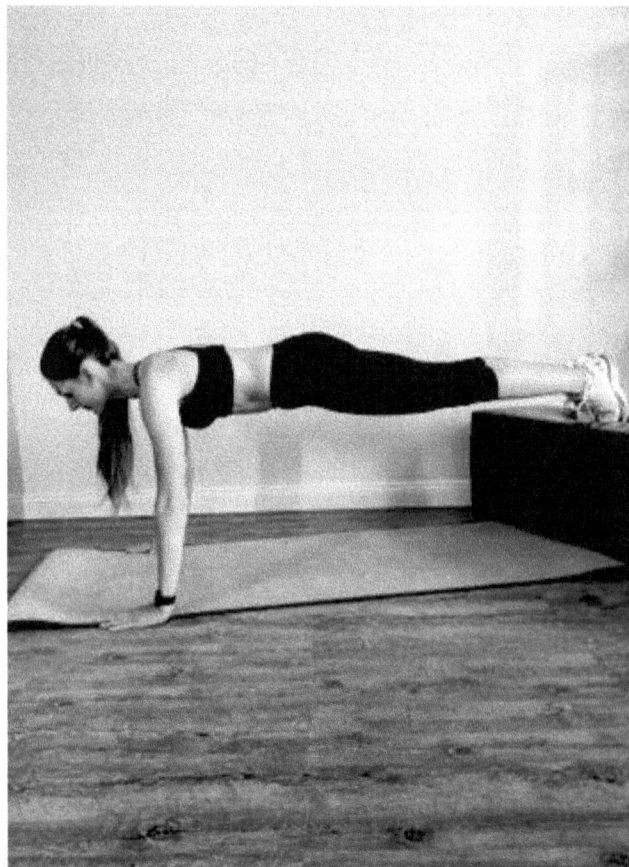

Dip

The main muscle being worked in this movement is your triceps (back upper arm); you will use a chair for this exercise.

Progression One – <u>Dips With Bent Legs</u>

Instructions

Sit on your chair or bench with your arms at your side and your feet flat on the floor, hip distance apart. Position your hands so that your palms are down beside your hips and have your fingers gripping the front of the chair.

Move your torso forward off the chair with your arms fully extended and your legs bent at 90 degrees. Slowly lower your butt down in a straight line until your arms are bent at 90 degrees, then push back up explosively to the starting position with your arms straight again.

Keep your back close to the chair throughout the entire movement.

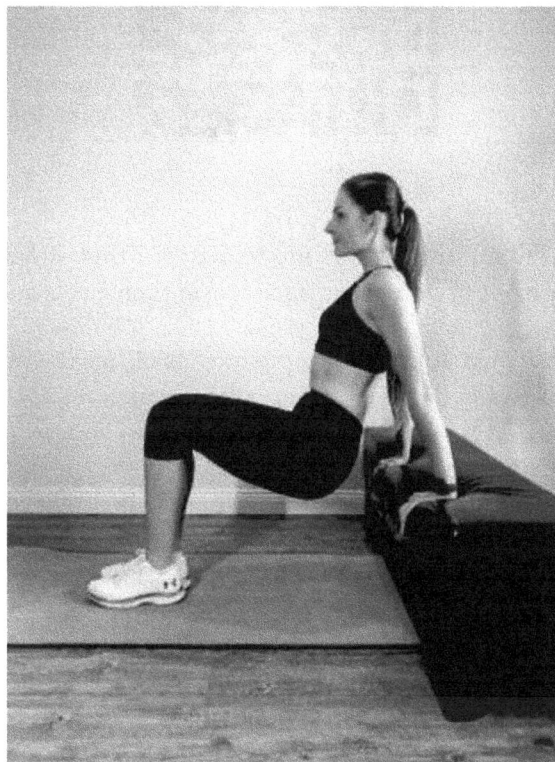

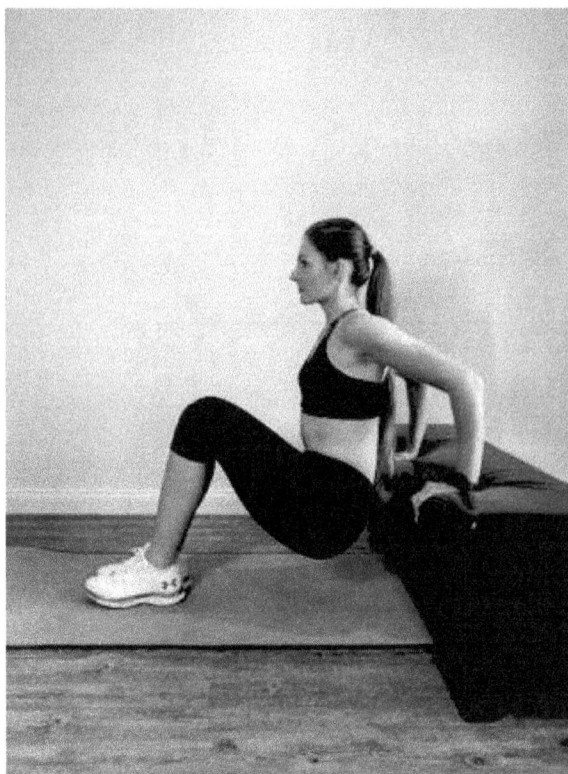

Progression Two – <u>Dips With Your Legs Straight</u>

Instructions

Focus on the same things as you did in the previous movement for this progression. The only difference here is that your legs will be straight in front of you with your feet on their heels and toes pointing to the ceiling.

Your arms will still bend to a 90-degree angle before pushing back up to the starting position while keeping your butt as close to the chair as possible throughout the movement.

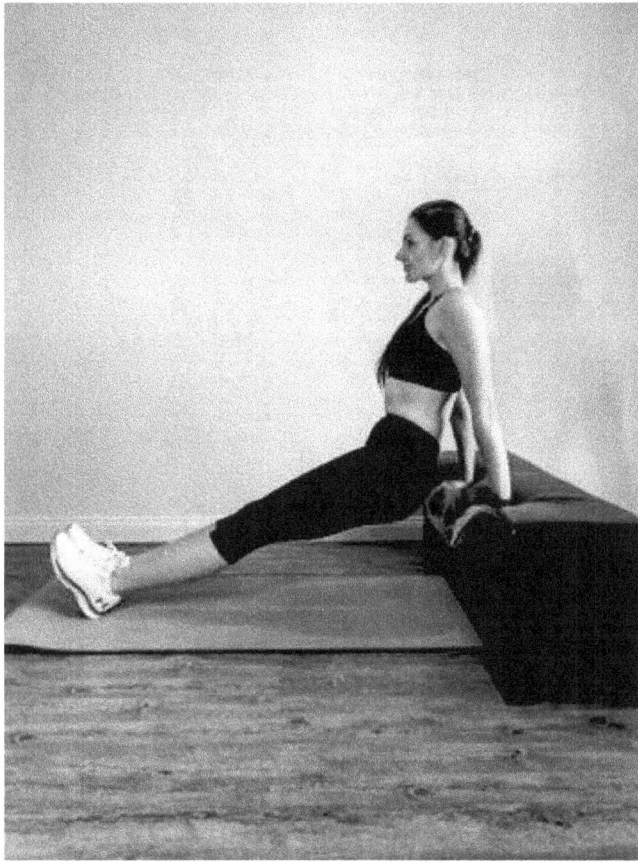

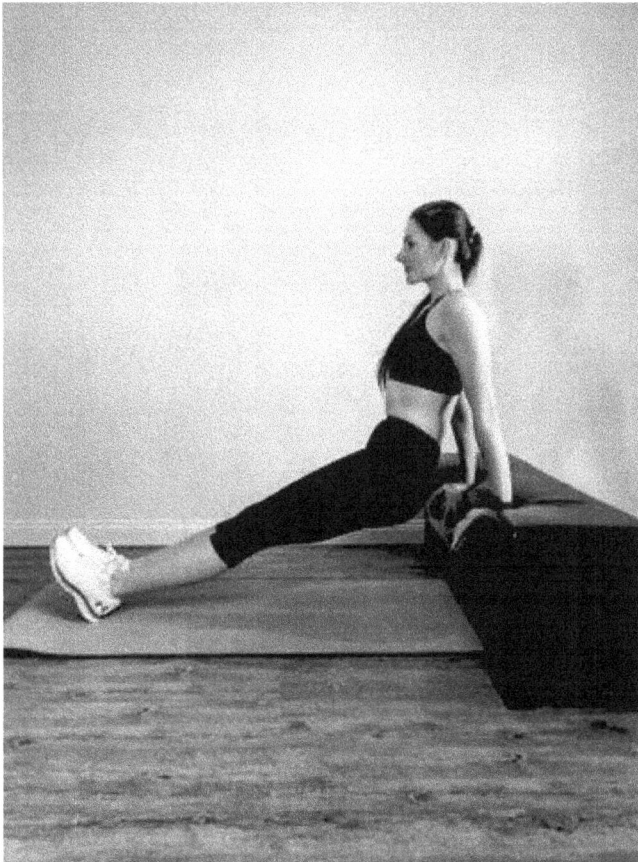

Progression Three- <u>Dips With Your Feet Elevated</u>

Instructions

The next progression and slightly harder variation of the chair dip will require 2 chairs. You will keep your legs straight with your feet on their heels and toes pointing to the ceiling for this one, but they will now be resting on a chair in front of you rather than the floor.

Everything else remains the same; your butt will stay close to the chair you are gripping with your hands, and you will lower yourself down by bending at the elbow until they are at a 90-degree angle before pushing up to the starting position with straight arms.

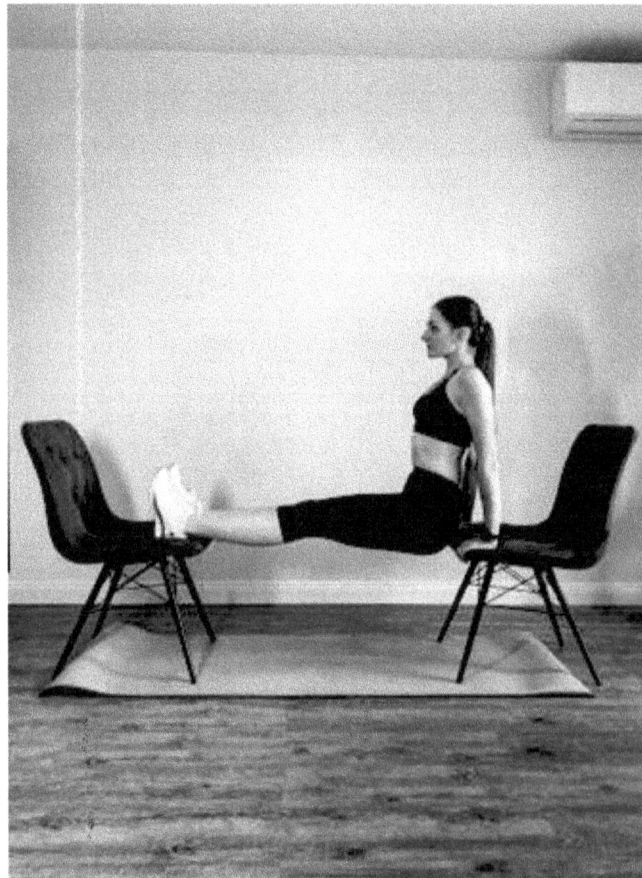

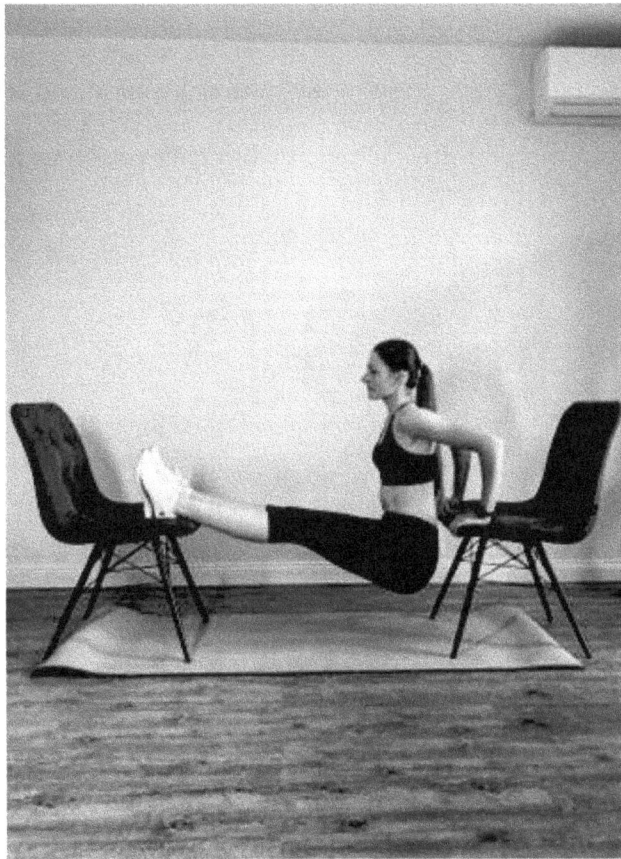

The Squat

The primary muscles used for this movement are the glutes (butt), the quads (front upper leg) and the hamstrings (back upper leg). The secondary muscles used are the calves and your core (lower back and stomach).

Progression one – <u>Standard Bodyweight Squat</u>

Instructions

Stand with your arms in a comfortable position, either reaching out straight in front of you or crossed over your chest. Have your feet shoulder-width apart with toes turned out slightly to open the hip joint.

Slowly lower your body by sticking your butt back until your thighs are parallel to the floor at 90 degrees or even slightly lower.

It's important to ensure your butt moves down and back, as this will keep your back straight and safe.

Pause at the bottom for a few seconds, then return to the starting position and repeat.

Stay on this progression until you can perform the reps by bringing your butt lower than 90 degrees, even as low as the top of your heels.

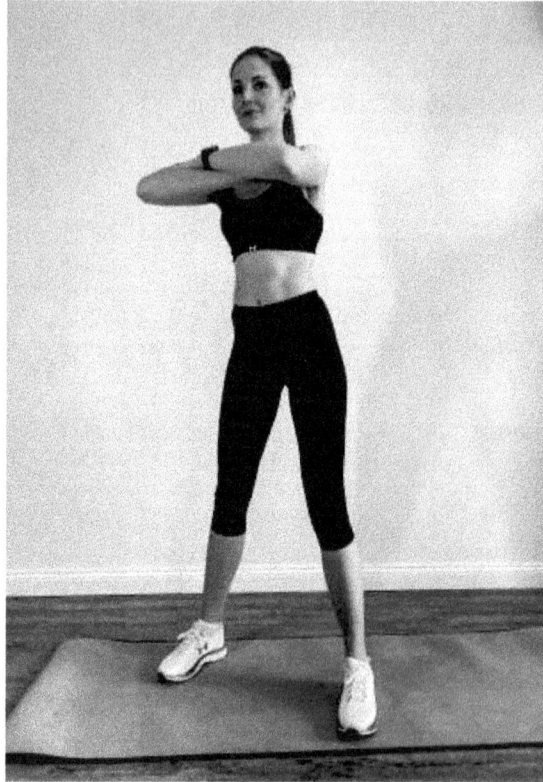

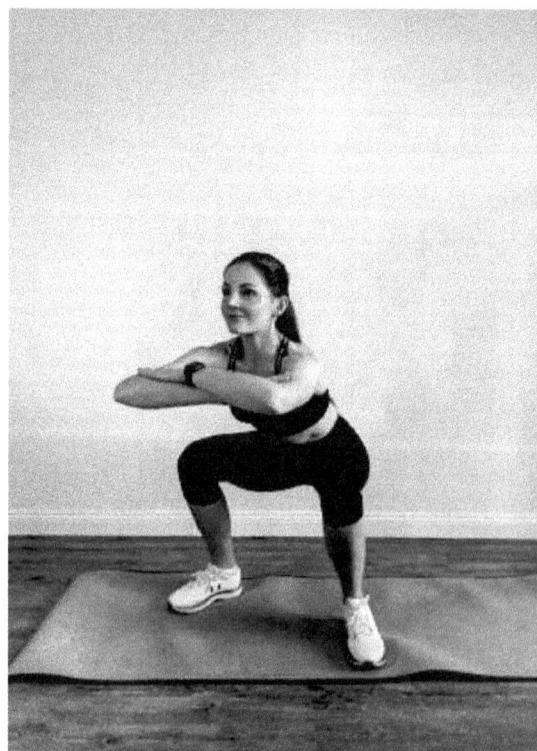

Progression Two - <u>Split Squat Lunge</u>

Once you have mastered the basic squat, you will move on to the split squat, the lunge. This exercise will put some more emphasis on balance and athleticism. This one will fire up the glutes, quads, calves, hamstrings, and core.

Instructions

Stand up straight with your feet hip-width apart and feet pointing straight. Begin by stepping forward with one foot while keeping both feet hip-width apart. Your hips, knees, and feet should all be in a straight line.

Slowly lower your torso towards the ground by dropping your hips until the knee on your back leg is about an inch from the floor, and then use your quad on your front leg to push your torso back up to the starting position.

 Repeat the prescribed number of reps before switching legs.

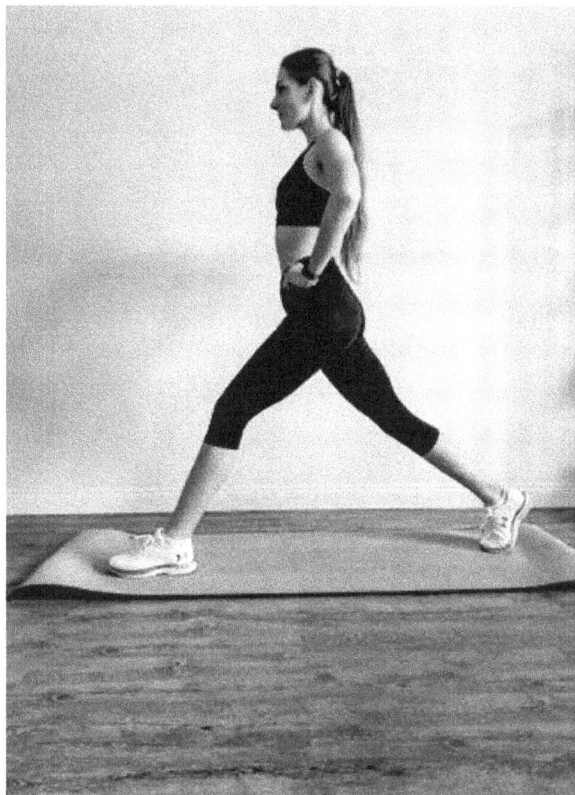

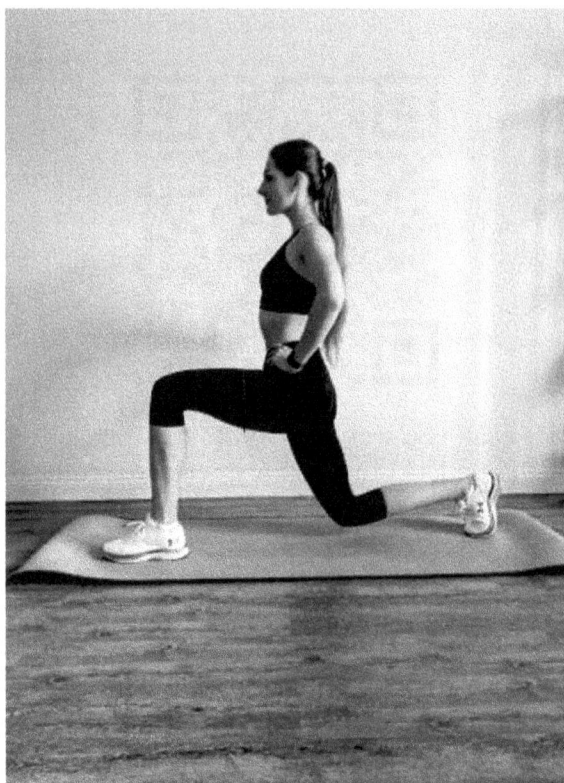

Progression Three - <u>Bulgarian Split Squat</u>

You might find this exercise quite a jump from the previous progression, but it shouldn't take you too long to get a handle on it. It works primarily on your quads (front upper leg) and your glutes (butt), but the great thing about this movement is you're working each leg individually as you will have your nonworking leg placed on a bench, chair, or your couch behind you.

If you have a weaker leg, then this will expose it. It will ensure you won't have your stronger leg compensating and taking most of the load, helping your weaker side as you might get when doing a regular squat. It will also test your balance, which is another thing that tends to get a bit shaky as we age, so it's a good idea to keep on top of it. This method is one of the best all-around legs exercises you can do, in my opinion.

Instructions

With one foot placed on a chair or couch behind you and the other foot on the floor out in front of you, you might need to hop your front foot out to get into the correct starting position, and you can set this up next to a wall if you need help for balance initially.

Begin by sinking slowly into a lunge/squat position until the front leg is parallel to the floor.

From here, explosively push up through your front heel straightening your front leg back up to a standing position and keeping your back leg stable on the chair behind you.

Continue for the prescribed number of reps on that leg before switching and repeating the exercise on the other leg.

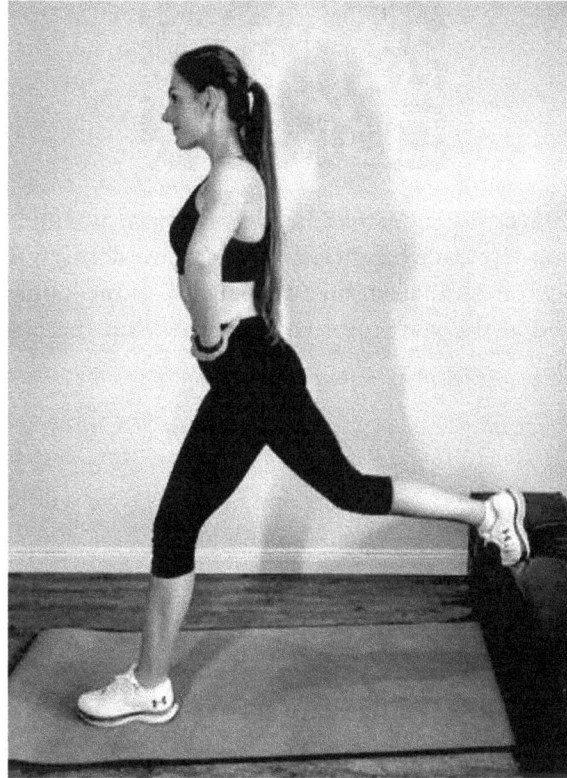

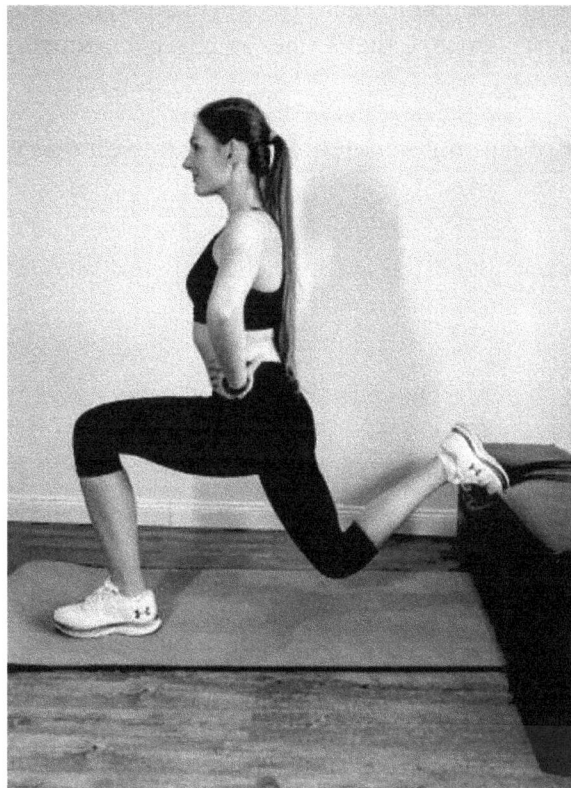

Progression Four - <u>Levitation Squats</u>

This progression is the toughest lower body exercise in the program. It will work the entire front and back of your legs and glutes and once again test your balance. I recommend doing this one next to a wall initially, as it will challenge every aspect of your physical strength and balance at the same time, so having your hand lean on a wall might be what's required at the start until you can build up the appropriate amount of strength to perform the exercise free standing.

Instructions

Start with one foot slightly in front of the other; from this position, you will lift your back foot off the ground slightly.

From here you will, you can have your arms stretched out in front of you for balance before slowly dropping your back knee to the floor while keeping that foot off the ground.

You will find that keeping your back foot off the floor will take away your ability to power up back to your standing position; it will feel a lot slower and more difficult.

This exercise is going to be a tough one and might take a while to get right, and if your back foot hits the ground at points throughout the movements, that's fine; as you get stronger and better at the movement, it will touch less and less.

Complete the prescribed number of reps on one leg before repeating on the other.

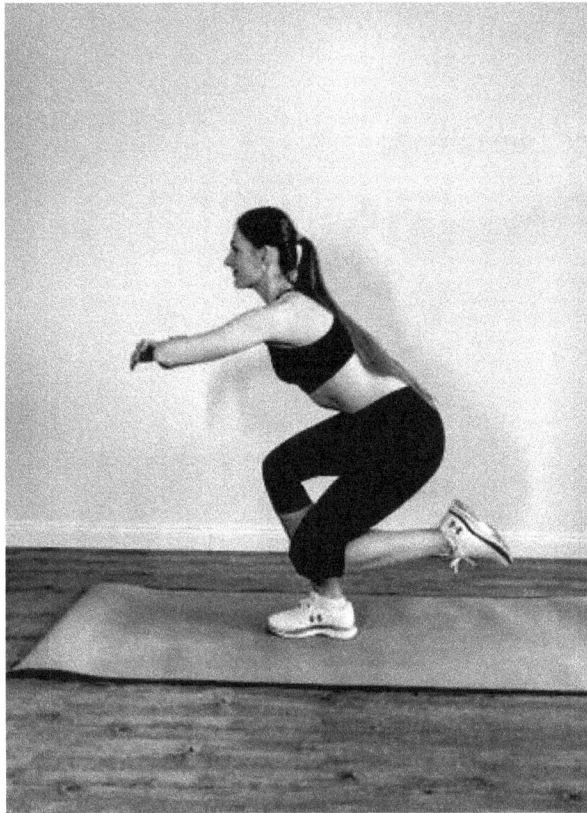

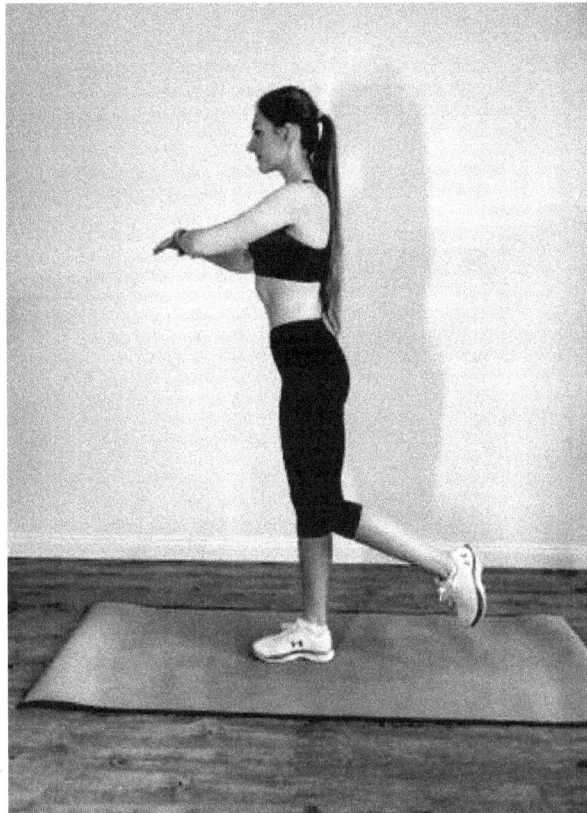

Hamstring and glute progression

Progression One – <u>Double Leg Glute Bridge</u>

This movement will focus on your glutes (butt) and the hamstrings (upper back leg). The secondary muscles used here will be your abs.

Instructions

To perform the double-leg glute bridge, lie on your back and place both feet on the floor; both legs should be bent at a 90-degree angle. Place your hands at your sides and then push through both heels evenly as you squeeze your glutes and lift your hips toward the ceiling.

At the top of the movement, your shoulders, hips, glutes, and knees should be straight.

Lower your glutes slowly and repeat the prescribed number of reps.

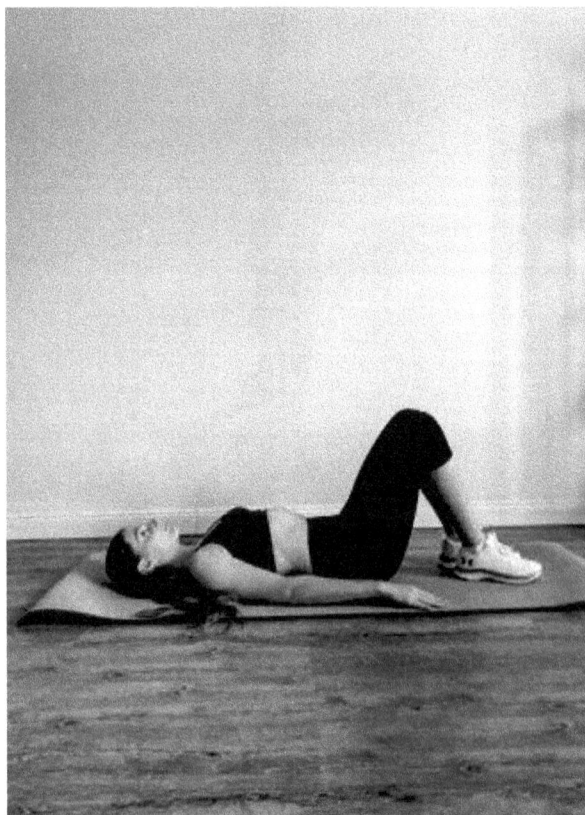

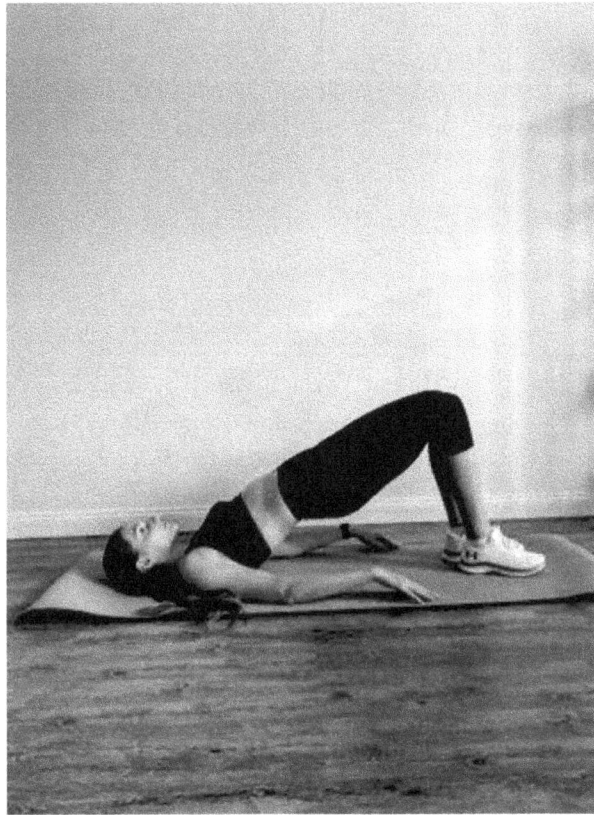

Progression Two – <u>Single Leg Glute Bridge</u>

Working the same muscles as the double glute bridge, this one takes it to a new level working each hamstring and each side of your glute individually, exposing any weaknesses in those areas.

Instructions

Begin like you did with the double-leg version, lie on your back and place your feet on the floor with your legs bent at 90 degrees. Place your hands out to your sides, palms resting on the floor.

From here, lift one foot off the ground straightening your leg and keeping it in line with the thigh of your other leg. It will remain in this position throughout the movement while your other leg works.

Now you will push through your heel as you squeeze your glutes and lift your hips upwards in a straight line with your torso. Lower your glutes slowly and repeat for the prescribed reps before switching to the opposite side.

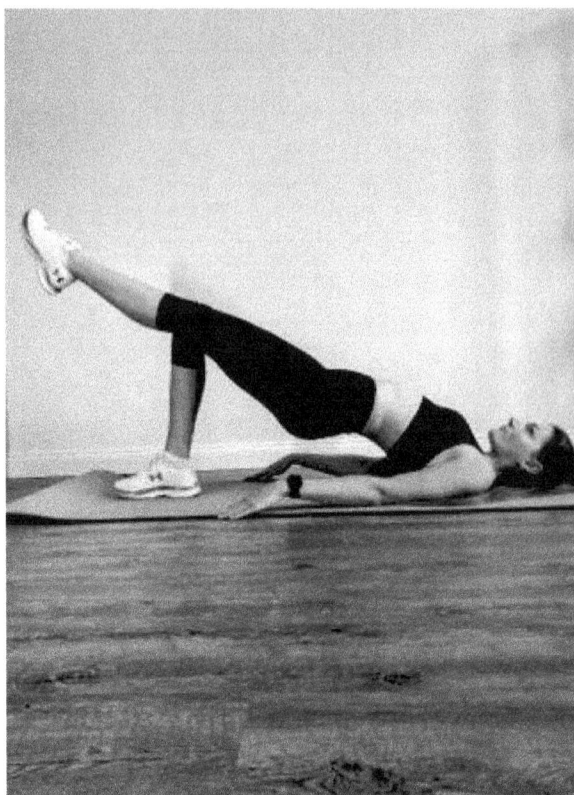

Progression Three - <u>Single leg Deadlift</u>

A great exercise overall, working many parts of the body. It will primarily work your hamstrings (back upper leg), glutes, lower back, and abs, but it will also test your balance and body control. This is one of the best movements you can do.

Instructions

Stand on one leg with your hands by your side while keeping your back straight, your shoulders back, and your core engaged. Begin to lean forward from the hips, not your waist.

Begin by leaning forward by bringing your hips back, keeping your front leg straight, and allowing your back foot to come off the ground behind you.

Keep your back leg straight as your foot comes up off the ground, and continue to lean forward as much as you can while keeping that back straight until you feel a stretch in your hamstring.

Return to your starting position by squeezing your glute muscle, and keep going for the prescribed number of reps before swapping sides.

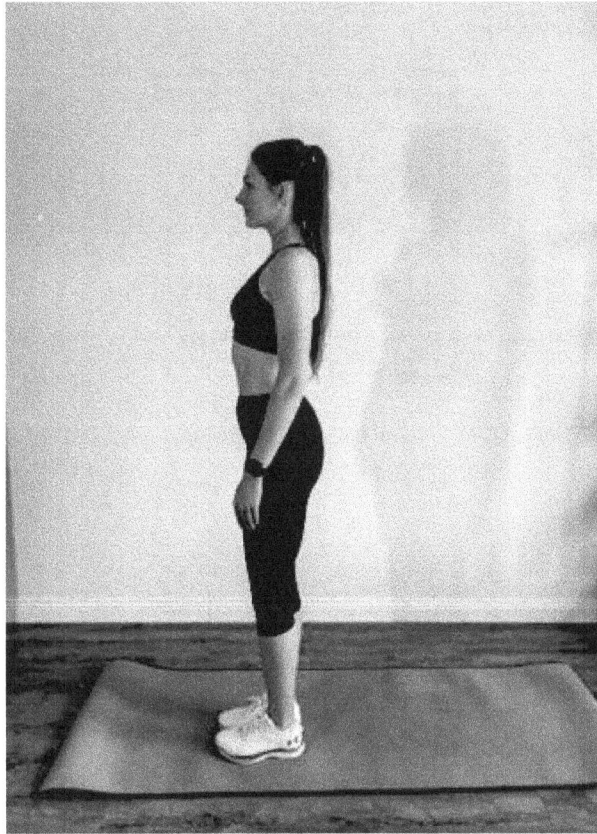

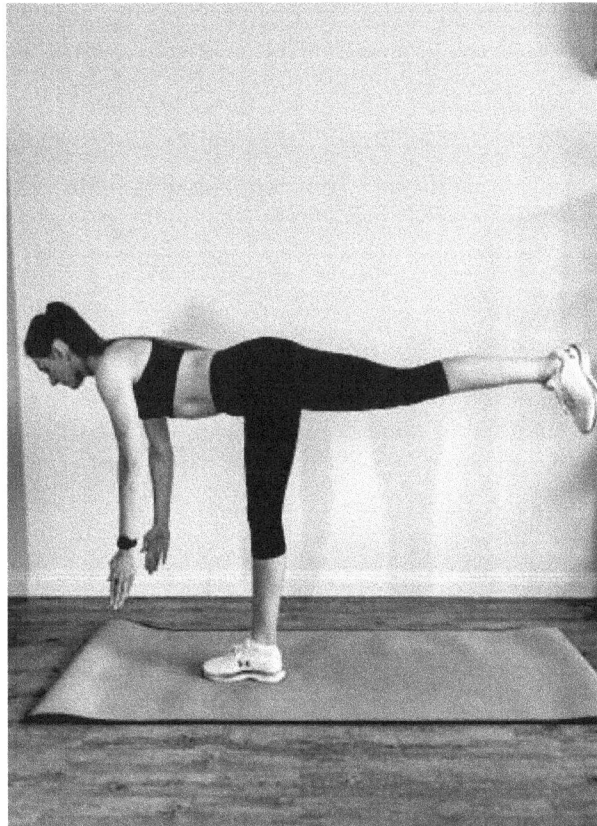

Pike progression

Progression One- <u>Push Away Pushups</u>

If this is too hard then try this variation – <u>push away pushups on knees</u>

Another variation of the pushup, but this one focuses on your shoulders and a little on your upper chest. You will also find your legs work during this one due to your legs being bent with your knees off the ground throughout the movement. It is a challenging but extremely effective exercise for building strong shoulders.

Instructions

Start down on the floor as if getting ready to do a pushup. Set up for this exercise by allowing your butt to travel back and up. You will keep your butt up the entire time while allowing your head to travel forward by bending at the elbow to 90 degrees before pushing back up and away to the starting position.

You will use your shoulders to press yourself away; if done correctly, you will feel this completely in the shoulders.

Ideally, your knees will be very slightly off the ground for the entire movement, but if you find this too challenging, you can keep your knees on the floor until you build up your strength.

Complete the prescribed number of reps.

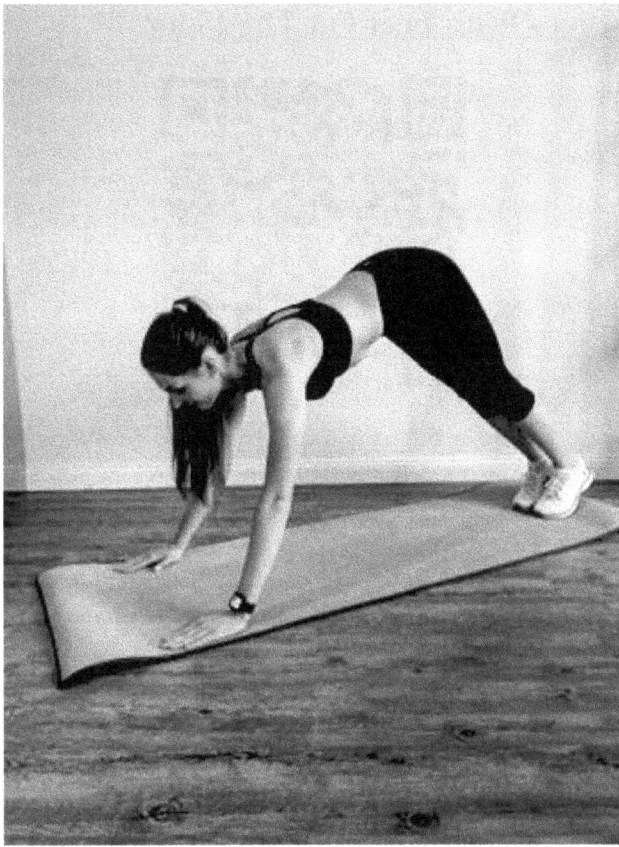

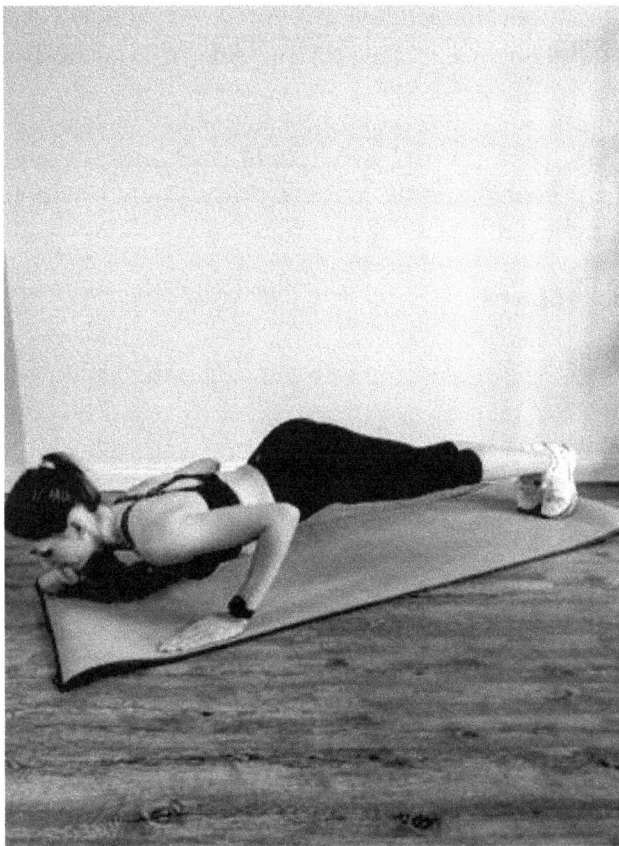

Progression Two - <u>Pike Press With Feet On The Floor</u>

An extremely difficult exercise and quite a bit of a jump from the previous progression. This one will take some practice and strength, but this isn't a race, so continue to be consistent with your training, and eventually, you will accomplish it.

This one will put your shoulders to the test but will also challenge the flexibility of your hamstrings, as you will need to keep your legs as straight as you can during the exercise. It will also hit your triceps (back upper arm) as a secondary movement.

Instructions

Position your feet on the floor, balancing on your toes with your hands shoulder-width apart and close enough to your feet so that your body forms an upside-down V position with the butt held high.

Without moving the rest of your body or bending at your knees, slowly bend your elbows to a 90-degree angle, be sure to keep your elbows slightly in towards the side of your body and not out in line with your shoulders.

Once your elbows are 90 degrees, push up explosively until your arms are straight, returning to the starting position. This movement is of a pressing motion, much like a push-up; however, you want to feel this in your shoulders and not so much your chest.

Repeat for the prescribed number of reps.

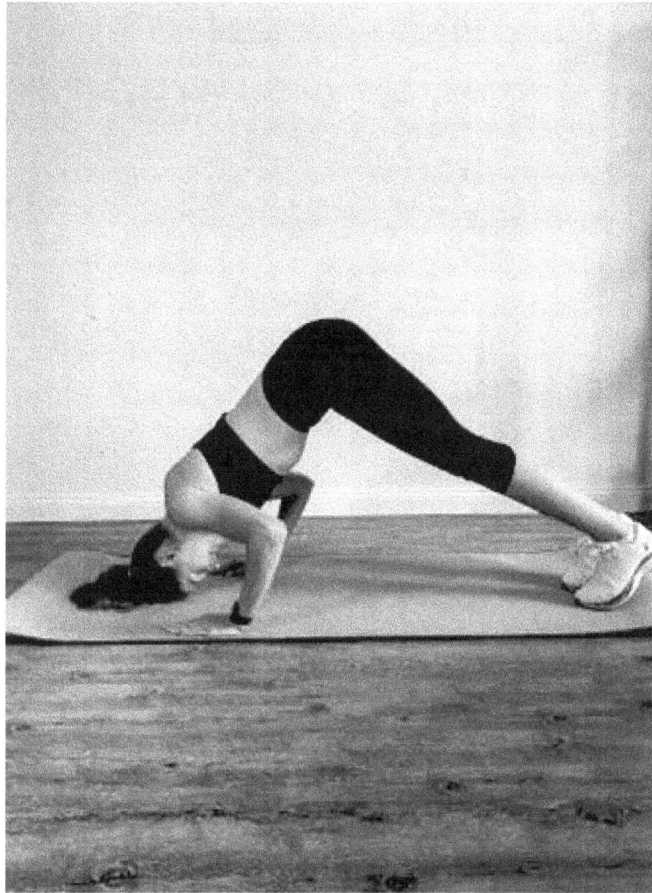

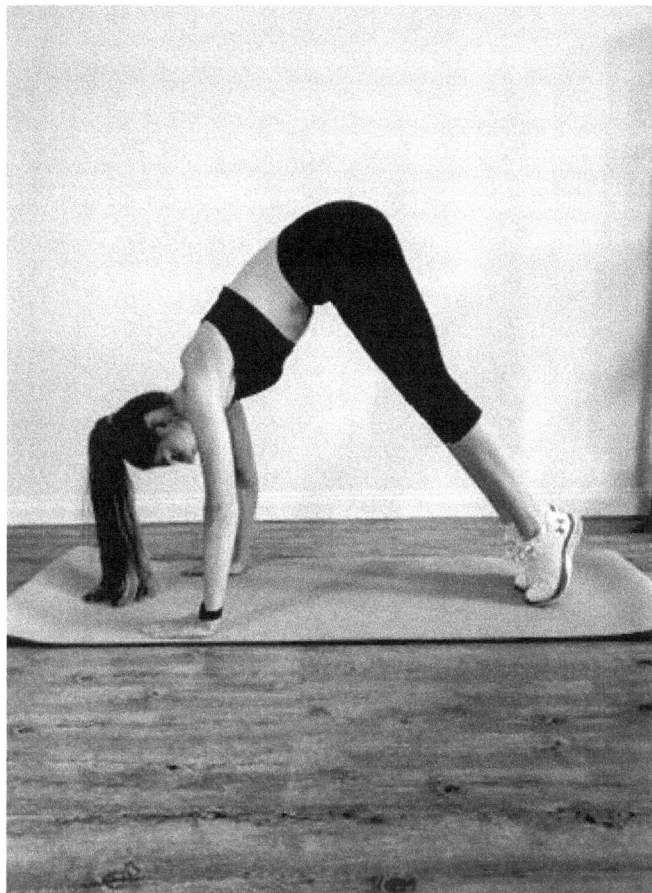

Progression Three – <u>Pike Press With Feet Elevated</u>

Instructions

This progression is the final of your shoulder-focused exercises; the pattern of the movement and the way you perform it is the same as the standard pike press, with the only difference coming from your feet being elevated off the ground on a step or chair.

All of the rules from the standard pike press apply, keep your legs as straight as you can, bend your elbows to 90 degrees with them slightly in towards the side of your body rather than out in line with your shoulders before pushing up.

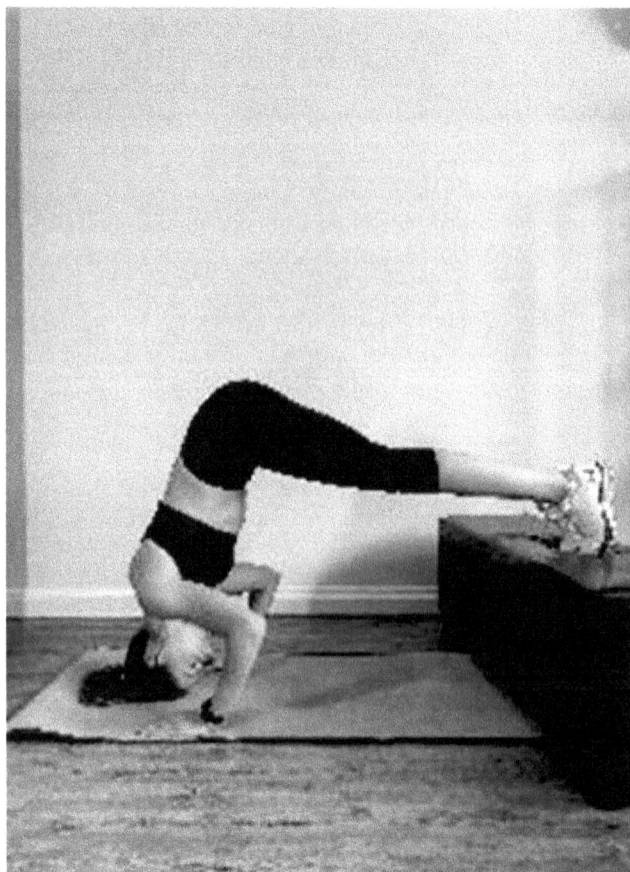

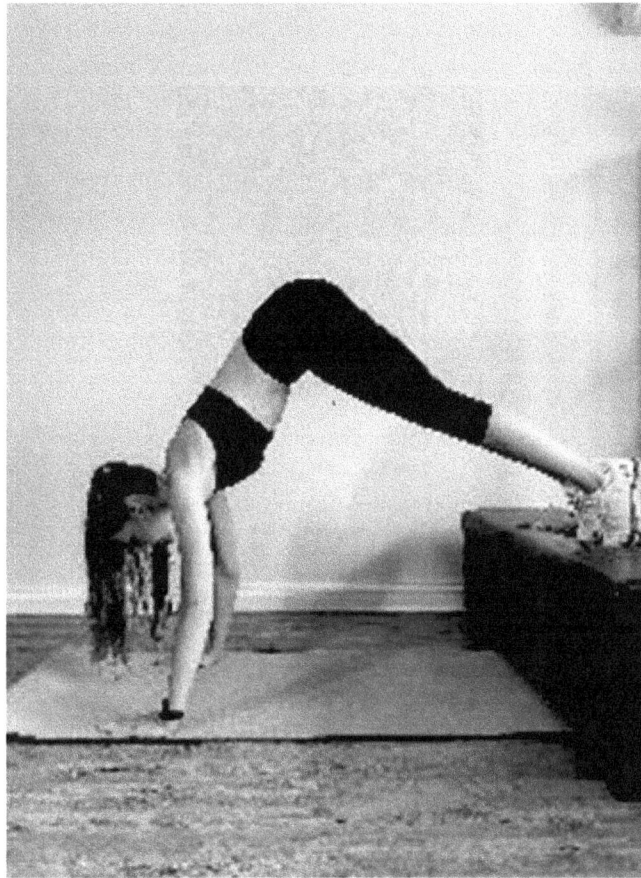

Other Exercises Included In This Program

Here are some other exercises included in the program that don't have progressions to them. You will build strength in these by adding reps to a certain extent but mainly by slowing down the speed at which you do the reps or pausing throughout the movements for longer periods.

Back

The back is a hard body part to work without some equipment, but here are a couple I have included in the program.

If it's affordable, I would highly recommend some type of suspension trainer like a TRX or one you can simply hook onto a door. You can do so many good bodyweights back exercises on them that could have you slowly work up to getting your first chin up.

I purchased one during covid and still use it now even though I have gym access again. TRX is the most well-known brand name and the best for suspension trainers, but plenty of more affordable versions of them can meet most budgets.

Suspension Trainer

TRX shop

For now, here are some great back exercises that you don't need any equipment for.

Back Widow

This exercise will work your upper back and rear deltoids (back of your shoulders).

Instructions

Lie on your back with your knees bent around 90 degrees and your feet flat. Bend your elbows and keep them tucked tight against your body. With your upper back flat against the ground, begin the exercise by driving your elbows down and back onto the floor.

The elbows obviously won't go anywhere since the floor is blocking them, but you should be able to push with enough force to lift your torso off the ground...using your upper back muscles, Lats, and rear shoulder muscles to do so. Pause at the top of the movement for a second before slowly lowering your torso to the ground and repeating for the prescribed number of reps.

Ensure you're lifting your torso by driving those elbows down rather than just trying to lift your shoulders off the ground. This movement would make it more of a sit, putting the focus on your abs rather than your back.

This exercise is one of the few in this program that doesn't have a progression, you could always put your feet on a step to make it harder, but you would want superior core strength to do this. For now, I would recommend you increase intensity firstly by adding more reps, then secondly by pausing at the top of the movement for a few seconds during each rep and slowing down the pace you perform each rep.

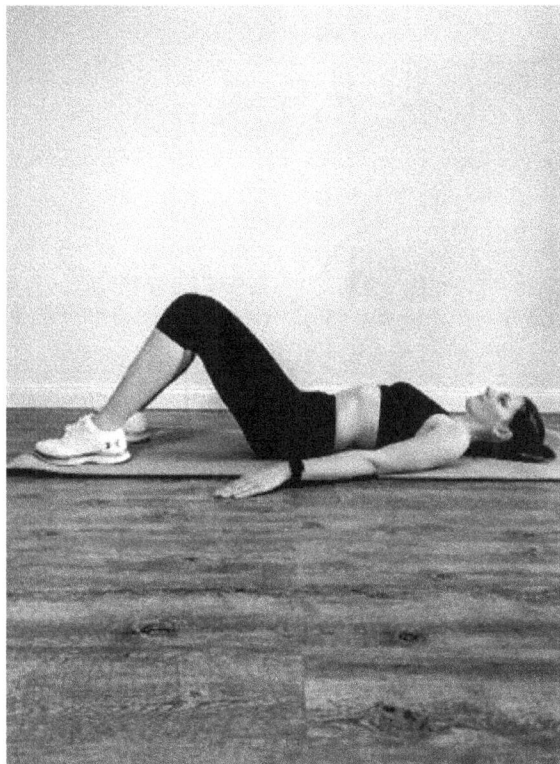

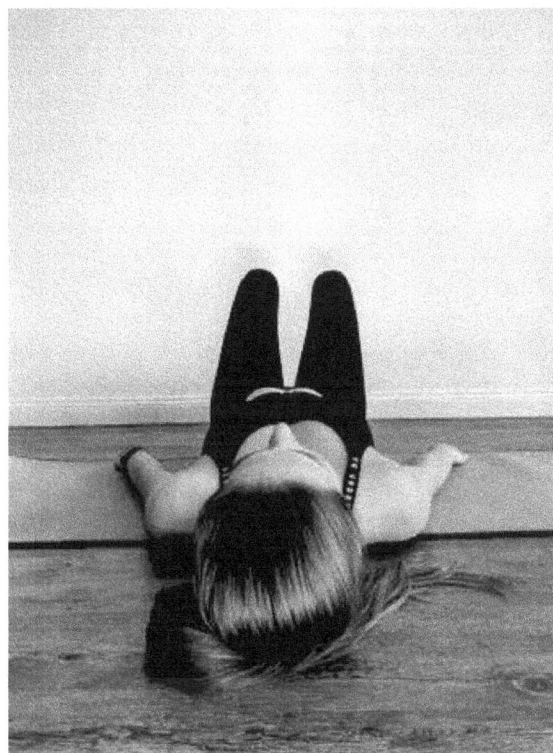

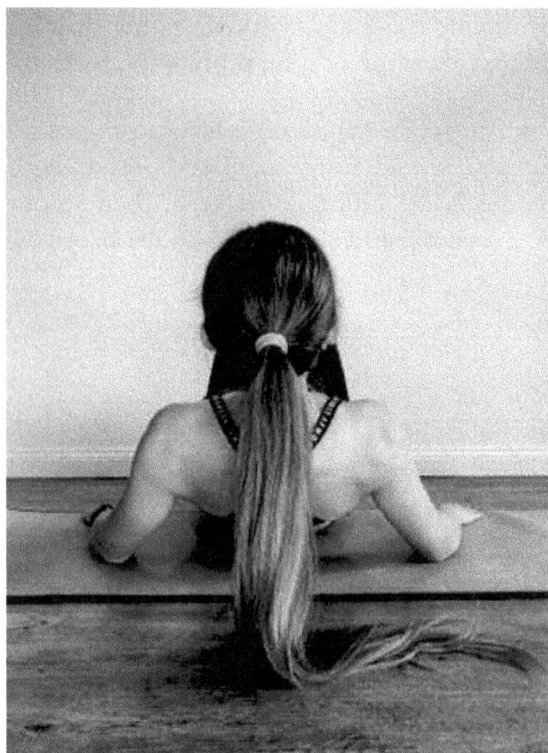

Door Jam Row

This exercise is great for your back and will have you working each side individually to expose any weakness and help increase your strength overall. It will work your biceps as a secondary muscle. All you needs is a regular doorway to do this exercise

Instructions

Position yourself in a doorway with your feet together and up against the side of the door frame (the left side of the doorway when working the right arm and vice versa). Have your working arm holding the inside of the door jamb.

Begin by dropping back and down (allowing your knees to bend as you do) until you're gripping arm is completely straight at the elbow.

From here, contract your biceps and pull yourself back up to a near-standing position by driving your elbow behind your body. Make sure you lead with the elbow and don't use your legs to push yourself back up.

Do the prescribed reps for one side of your body before moving to the other.

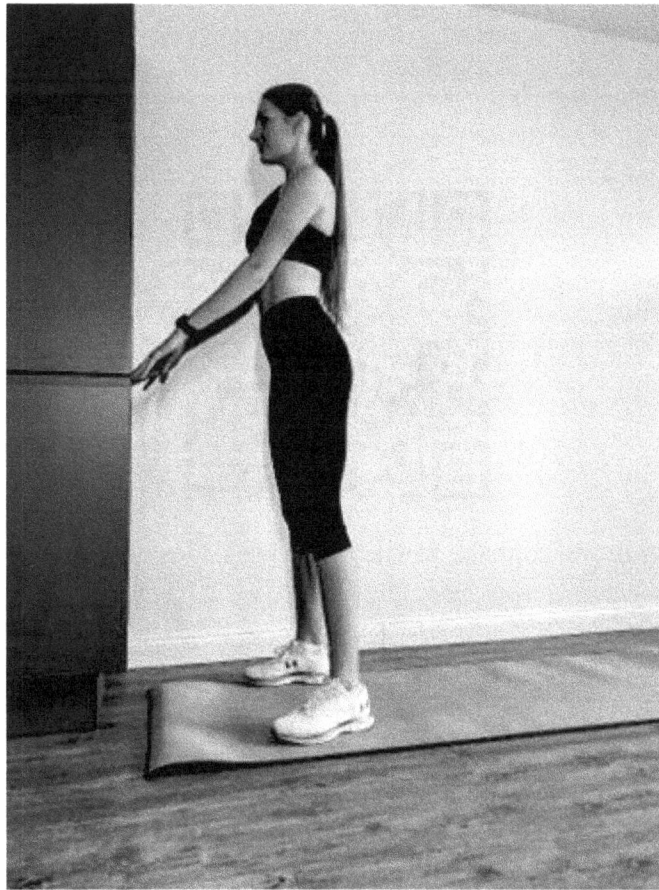

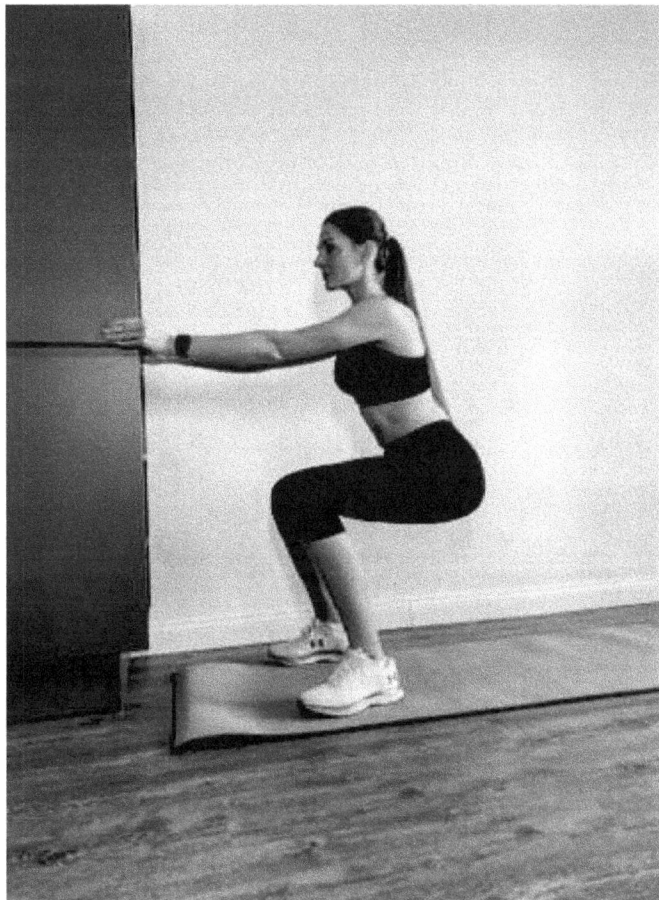

Core

Heel taps

A great core exercise bringing more emphasis to your obliques (sides of your stomach and love handles) than a normal crunch or sit-up.

Instructions

Lay on your back, have your knees bent and your arms at your sides with your back and feet flat on the floor. Raise your shoulders off the floor and to the left while reaching out with your left arm to touch your left heel; hold it there for a second before slowly returning to the starting position and moving to the right side.

Continue to alternate between left and right with each rep.

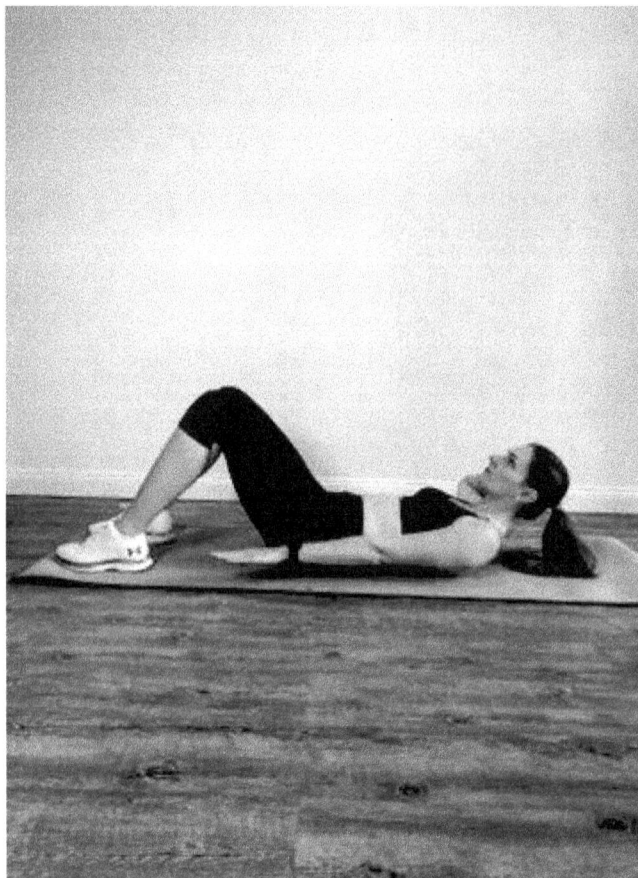

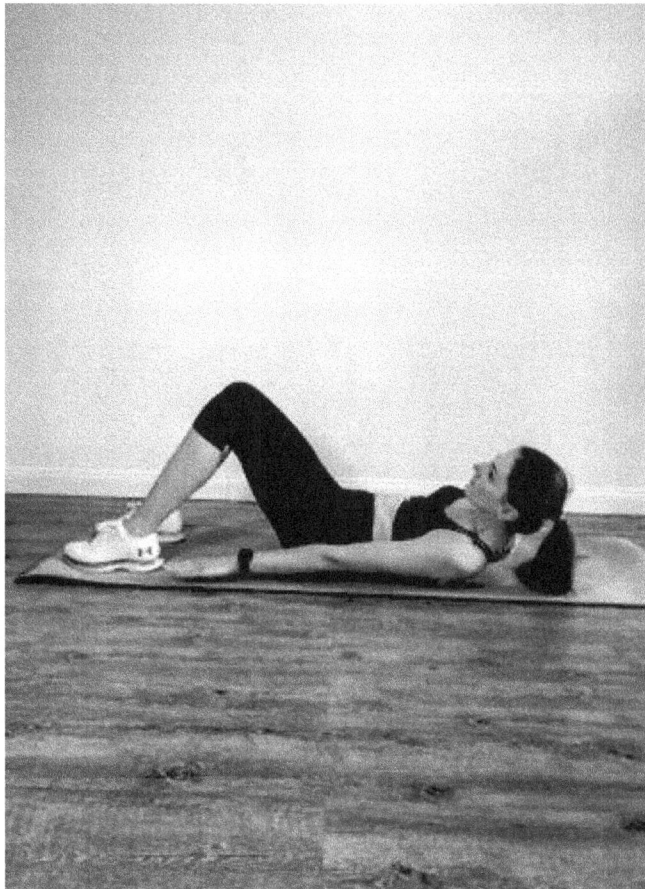

Supermans

Supermans are a great exercise for your entire core but, more specifically, the often neglected lower back. Do not swing through the movement to ensure you get the most out of this one. Keep in control of your body the entire time. It's not as easy as it might look.

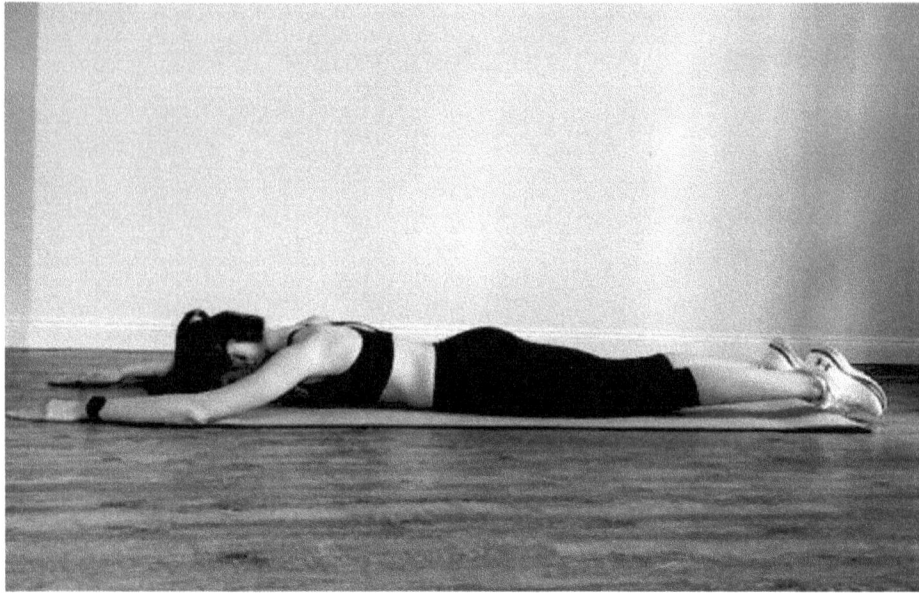

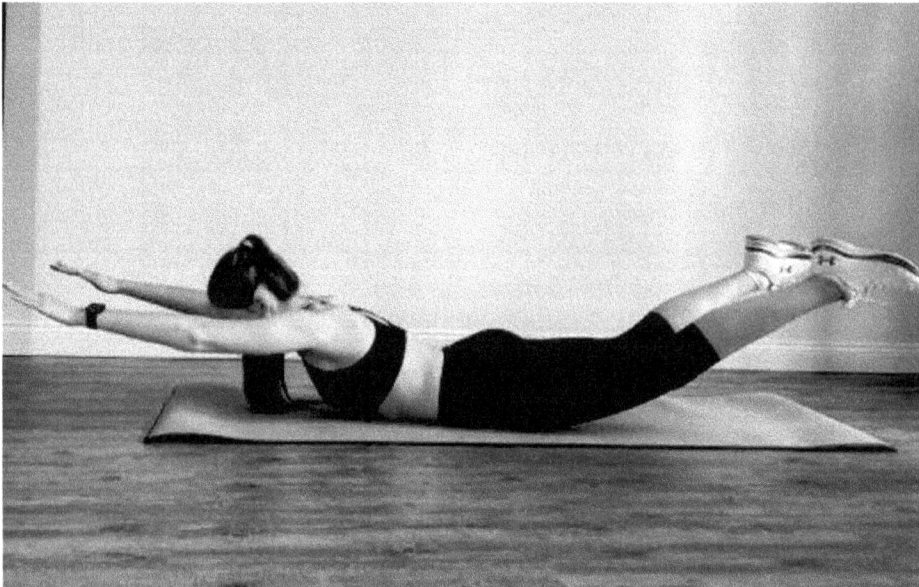

Instructions

Begin by lying face down on a mat or the floor with your arms and legs stretched like Superman. Raise both arms and both legs off the ground at the same time, leaving your stomach and hips on the ground; hold it for a second, then release back down to the starting position. Keep your arms and legs straight throughout the entire set. Repeat for the prescribed number of reps.

Side plank

A great overall core exercise, this will focus on the static strength of your entire core, hitting many of the smaller muscles that might not get the love they deserve during many of the more popular core exercises you see. It will also test your shoulder strength and balance, working each side individually.

Instructions

Begin by lying on your side, resting on your elbow; make sure your elbow is in line with your shoulder, and have your legs out straight with your feet stacked on each other.

From here, lift your hips off the ground to rest on your elbow, forearm, and the sides of your feet. Your body should be kept in a straight line off the ground, your hips will want to dip towards the ground, but this is where those abs need to kick in to maintain a straight position.

Remember to ensure your resting elbow is directly under your shoulder. Hold it there, and remember to breathe throughout the movement.

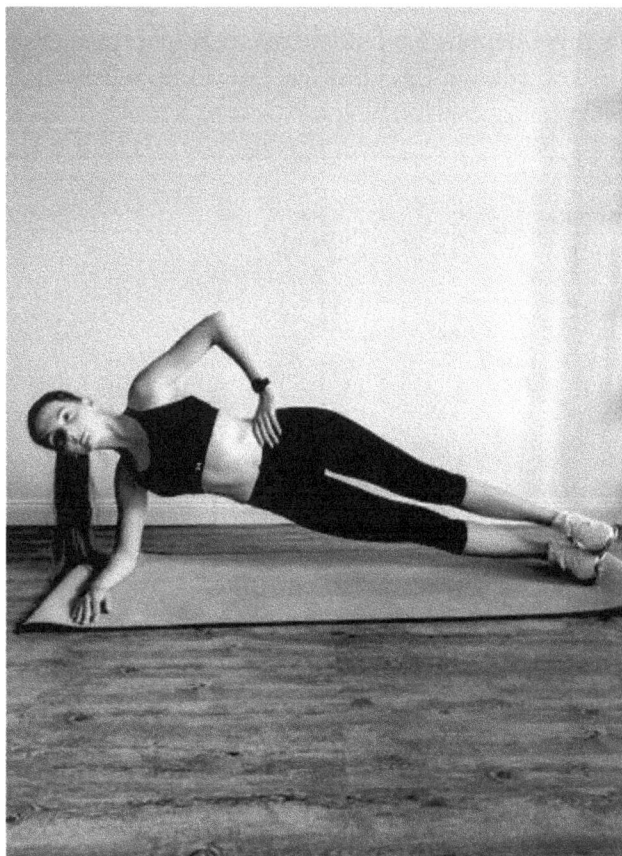

Legs

Sumo squat

A similar movement to the normal squat with a few slight differences will bring the focus towards your inner thigh rather than the front and back of your legs. As with most compound leg exercises you have done already, it will also work your glutes.

Instructions

Stand with your feet wider than your shoulders and your toes pointing outwards with your arms positioned wherever is the most comfortable, either crossed over your chest or stretched out in front of you.

Keeping your chest and core engaged, push your hips back and bend at your knees, lowering your body until your thighs parallel the floor. If done correctly, you will feel a nice stretch on your inner thighs, pause for a second and then return to the starting position. Continue for the prescribed number of reps.

There are no progressions with this one, but I would advise that as it gets easier, you fill up a backpack and wear it to add extra resistance, or you could always buy a set of dumbbells to hold.

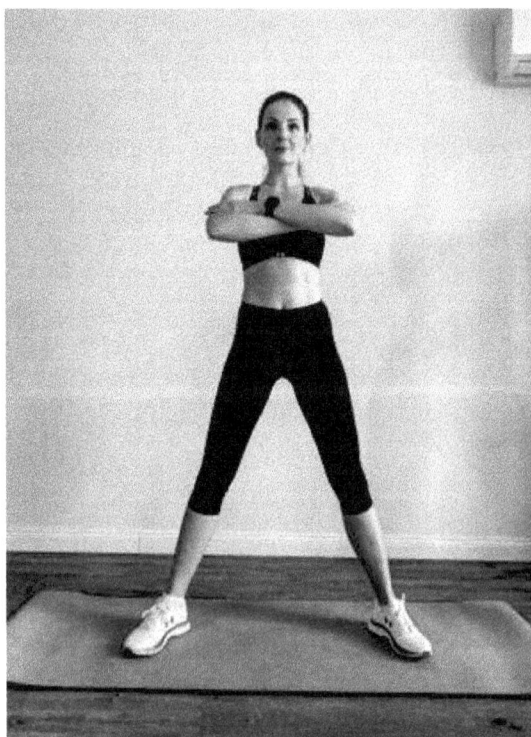

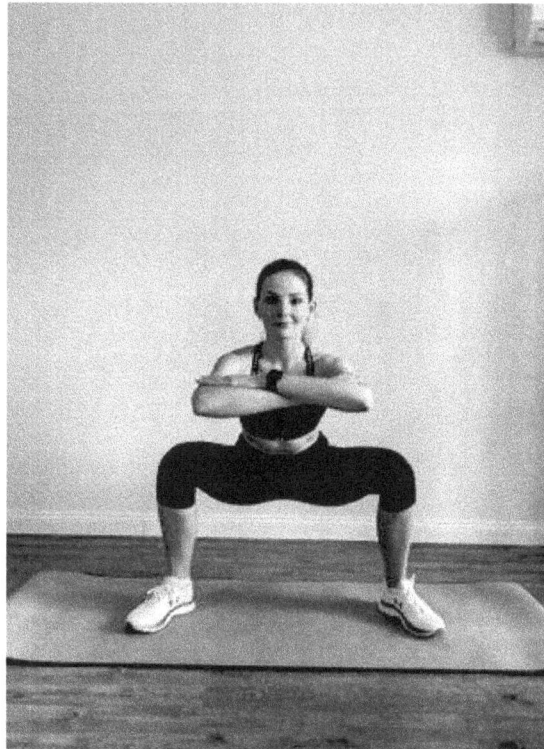

Fire hydrants

This exercise might look easy when you watch it, but for those of us with tight hips, you will feel the challenge when performing it. It's a great exercise to open up the hip joint, which is often active and tight due to our lack of daily movement and sitting at a desk for much of the day.

Instructions

Begin by getting down on your hands and knees with your legs hip-width apart and your hands on the floor directly under your shoulders. While squeezing your core and keeping your arms completely straight, lift one leg outwards to a 45-90 degree angle while maintaining the bend in that leg and without moving the rest of your body.

Repeat the prescribed number of reps before switching legs.

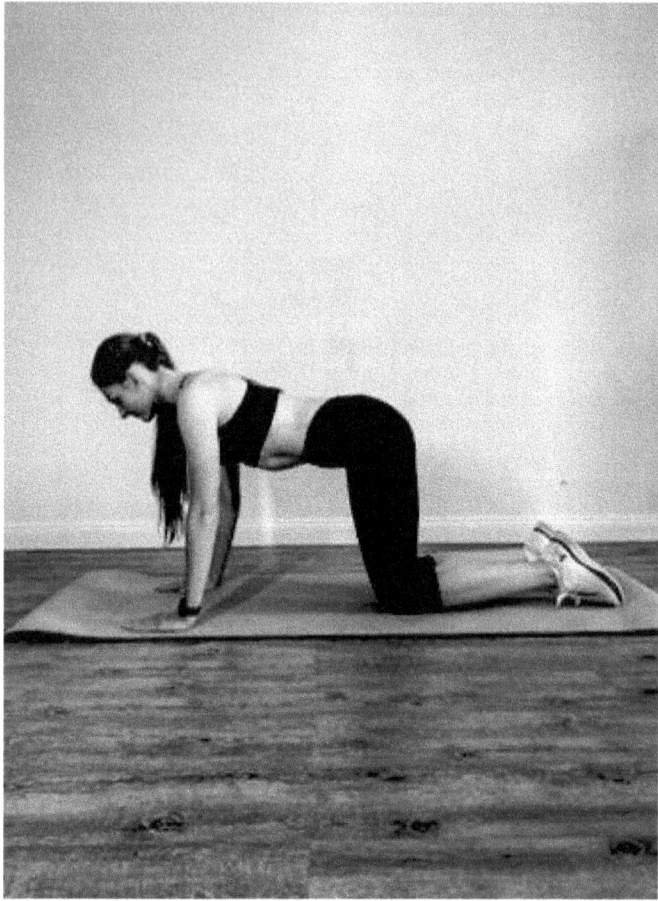

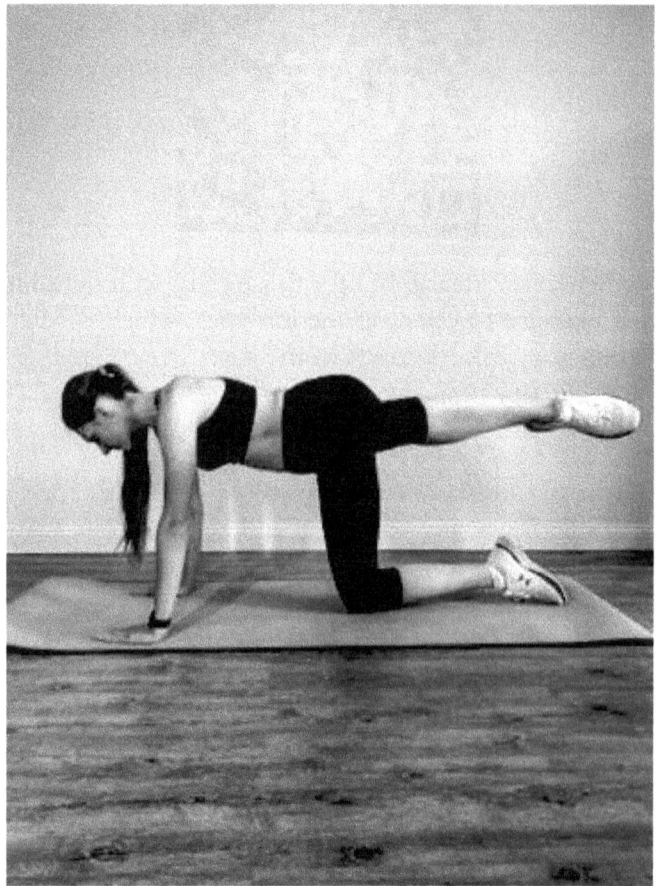

Step ups

A great functional movement that can be used to build strength, balance, and cardio depending on the pace at which you perform the movement. This movement will work your glutes, quads, calves, core, and hamstrings.

Instructions

Begin by standing straight in front of a step, bench, or chair. Choose something that has enough height that will challenge you but at the same time keep you safe as far as your balance goes. Maybe begin by doing it next to a wall so you can lean your hand against it for stability until your confidence grows.

Find your balance on your lead foot and lift the other leg up, placing your foot on the bench in front of you; make sure your foot is completely flat, and push through your heel, lifting your body until you're standing on the bench with both feet flat.

Return to the starting position and repeat for the prescribed number of reps on the same leg before switching over.

For an extra challenge, wear a backpack with some weight or keep your nonworking foot off the bench at the top of the movement throughout the entire set.

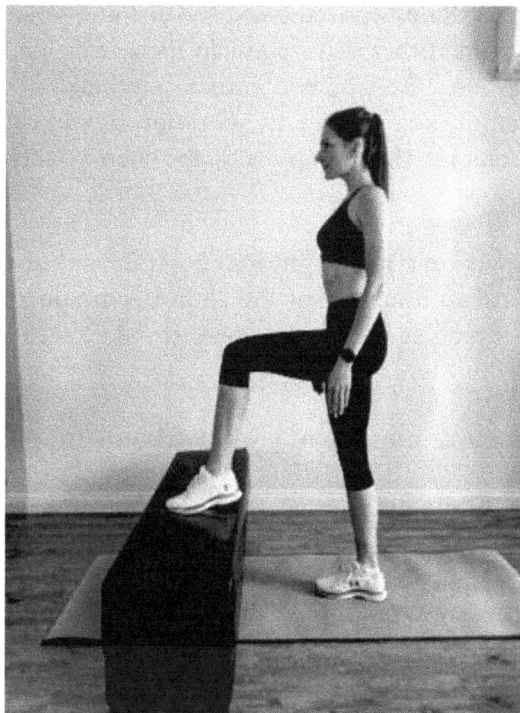

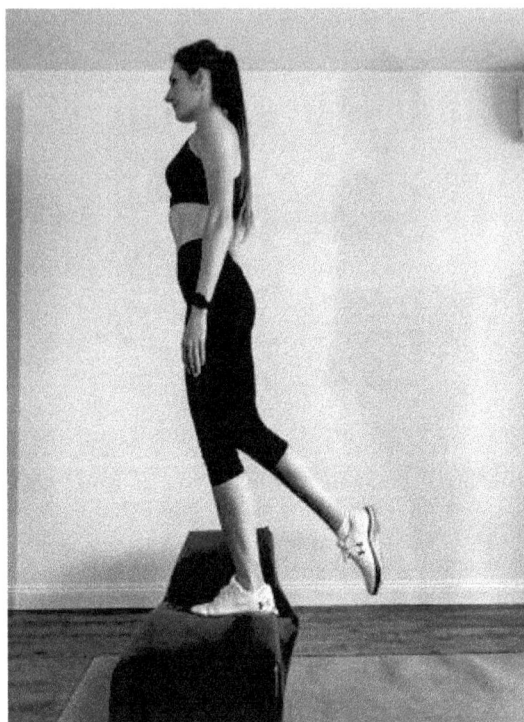

The Only Cardio You Will Ever Need

The only cardio you need to be doing in this program is walking, unless you're an athlete or play a sport that requires you to be fit in a specific type of cardio movement like running, then walking is all you need for good health, a good body and to increase longevity.

As mentioned earlier, 8000-10,000 steps per day is your goal. For good heart health, 8000 should be the minimum you aim for, and a fair chunk of that count can be made up with your non exercise activities thermogenesis (NEAT). These are the steps you take just performing your everyday activities like shopping, cooking, or playing with the kids. Some other ways you can increase your NEAT are parking a little further away from work or getting off the bus a stop or two earlier and walking the rest. One thing I like to do is make sure I walk around in between my sets during my workout instead of just sitting like I see most people do. You will be surprised at how quickly these steps add up when you find creative ways to increase your NEAT.

Your NEAT has a much bigger impact on your weight loss goals than your actual workouts; think about it, on workout days, you only spend around an hour out of the 24 hours in your day exercising; that's not much, so if you spend the rest of your time sitting at a desk it's going to take you longer to cut the fat than someone that is constantly on the move.

What you do and how much you move outside of your workouts matter.

If you want to go beyond just heart health and put an indent into your weight loss goals, then push your step count up to 10,000 per day. Remember this is an average over your entire week; you will find some days you move a little less while other days you move more than usual, which will make up for it, so don't stress if you don't reach your step count every day; sometimes life just gets in the way.

I have added a 30-45 minute walk on your off days for this program to help you hit your step count. Walking has many benefits beyond burning calories and helping you look good. I think its positive effects on your mental health far outweigh the rest of the benefits. Getting outside in the fresh air, getting some vitamin D that most people are deficient in, and clearing your head from daily stress makes walking such a powerful thing for your overall wellbeing.

Rucking

Want to take your walking game to the next level for added calorie burn and fitness? Try rucking.

What is rucking, you might ask? Rucking is simply adding resistance to your body while you walk. A few companies sell backpacks, weight plates, and vests specifically designed for rucking, but this can also be achieved by simply filling a backpack with whatever you can find to add a certain amount of weight and wearing it while you walk.

Rucking has been shown to burn slightly fewer calories than running without the damage that running does to your joints, so I highly recommend it for your daily walk.

Chapter 6:

A Quick Word on Nutrition

As far as your nutrition goes, my philosophy is that you can follow whatever diet plan you like so long as you think you can stick with it long-term. There are many diets out there to choose from, such as Keto, paleo, or flexible dieting; they all work, but none of them are magic; the one thing they all require for you to lose weight is you need to be eating at a caloric deficit. Without the calorie deficit, you won't lose weight however choosing the right deficit is important if you take out too many calories; you will crash your metabolism, mess up your hormones, and have no energy.

I will go through the basics here, but as mentioned at the beginning of this book, I have a free nutrition guide; I urge you to download and put it to good use. It's got everything you need to know to fix your nutrition and ensure your success. Download it here.

I prefer flexible dieting as I don't want to completely cut out any macronutrients together, nor do I want to give up some of the not-so-healthy treats I enjoy. As long as you get the portion sizes right, then I feel they all have their place in a healthy diet. I know many people who do Keto and have sustained it long-term with great results, so there is no right or wrong way; it's purely a matter of personal preference and what will work best with your lifestyle.

I heavily lean towards intermittent fasting as a great tool to implement regardless of your diet. When I'm eating at a caloric deficit and dividing fewer calories out between the standard 3 meals and 2 snacks over a whole day, I find that my meals end up being way too small to keep me satiated.

This made it harder to stick to long term as I was hungry all day and constantly waiting for my next meal. The other thing that you will find with a conventional 5-6 meal a day plan is that you need to spend a large amount of time meal prepping for days ahead of time to always have your next meal ready when you need it. I still meal prep a bit, but not to the same extent I did when eating more regularly throughout the day; it's unnecessary. I want to make my life easier, not harder.

Intermittent fasting allows you to give up living out of Tupperware containers every day and eat more of your food fresh as it's cooked since you're eating fewer meals daily. The great thing about it is that those meals can be larger in quantity since you are condensing those 5-6 smaller meals into 2-3 larger meals, making them more enjoyable and fully satisfying.

Plus, there are so many other health benefits that come along with intermittent fasting other than weight loss, such as cognitive function and hormone balance, just to name a few.

I recommend looking into it and seeing if it's something you might like to try. If it's not your thing, don't stress; intermittent fasting is merely a tool I use. It certainly doesn't determine your success or failure in losing weight and building a great body. That is determined by your consistency in eating at a caloric deficit and speeding up your metabolism by adding lean muscle and building strength.

Your Magic Number

I know the title of this book focuses on the workout plan, but let's face it nutrition holds the key to transforming your body. If you don't give it the attention it deserves, the workout, while making you strong, won't change how your body looks. If your body fat levels are too high, you won't see any of the newly toned muscles you have built through working out; that comes down to how you eat.

In this section, you will learn how to calculate the individual calorie number that you should be taking in on a daily basis. I understand that counting calories isn't for everyone, it takes time, and it's another chore you need to add to your day, so I will also show you another method you can use to make life easier if you are dead set against counting calories.

Let's begin with some nutrition basics, and il try to keep it short.

Let's start with calories and macronutrients or macros, as they are commonly referred to as these are two terms that get thrown around a lot when it comes to dieting. A calorie is a unit of energy we need to fuel our body. To lose weight, you need to be burning off more of those units of energy than you take in; whatever is left over gets stored as body fat.

Macros, on the hand, are what calories are made of. The three macros that make up calories are proteins, carbohydrates, and fats, and all three serve different bodily purposes.

From calorie value, there are 4 calories in every gram of carbohydrate and protein and 9 calories in grams of fat.

Each of the three macronutrients plays a specific role in your body; when you set out to improve your health and transform your body, you need to look beyond just total calories so that you can get the most out of your nutrition not only with how you look but also energy levels and health and wellness.

Let's start with protein

Protein is found in every part of your body, from your organs, tissues, hormones, and, of course, your muscles; it's made up of amino acids; these amino are essential not only when it comes to building strength and lean muscle but also helping you hold on to that muscle while you are in your weight loss phase.

Protein repairs your body from the resistance training you do, which is what this program is about. Most people don't get anywhere near enough protein in their diet, and if you exercise regularly, you need more than those who don't. One of the benefits of protein you might not know is that it has the highest thermic effect on food, meaning it requires more energy (calories) to digest it than other macronutrients. You won't have to aim for Anything between 0.82 – 1.3G of protein per pound of body weight daily. The higher level is for, the more active strength athletes that carry a good amount of muscle. For someone starting, I would stick to 0.82.

The following is a list of protein sources to include in your diet.

Very Lean	Fairly Lean	Very Fatty
Eat regularly	**Eat a few times a week**	**Eat occasionally**
Egg whites	Whole eggs.	Ribeye steak
	Flank steak	Pork spareribs
Nonfat ricotta		
	Chicken thigh, skinless	Top sirloin
Chicken breast, skinless	Trimmed brisket	Chicken, with skin
Turkey breast, skinless	Turkey leg, skinless	Porterhouse / New York
	Trimmed stewing beef	Sausage / chorizo
Pork tenderloin		
	Turkey bacon.	T-bone steak
Pork chop	Beef shank	Salami
Cottage cheese	Burger patties	Filet Mignon
	Lean sausage	-80% lean ground beef
Tofu		
	80% lean ground beef	Beef / pork / lamb ribs
Bone broth	Beef jerky	Salmon filet, with skin
Deli beef/ham/turkey	Bison.	Beef short ribs
	Salmon filet, skinless	Canned fish in oil
Oysters		
	Full-fat yogurt.	Beef tri-tip
Crab/Lobster	Canned sardines	Lamb shank
93% Lean ground beef	Full-fat ricotta.	Bacon / Pork belly
	Lamb chop	Hot dogs
95% Lean ground turkey		
	Cheeses.	
Turkey jersey	Lamb leg	
		(Also, any meat with a lot of
Kangaroo	Whole milk.	*untrimmed fat or skin)*
	Pork sirloin	
Venison		
	Round / rump steak	
Protein powder	Leg ham	
Non yogurt		
Shrimp/prawns		
Mussels		
Scallops		
Tuna/canned in water		
White fish		

Meats are the most common source of protein, but it isn't your only option; there are many plant-based foods that are good sources of protein and leaner in calories at the same time. Ensuring you get some of your protein from non-animal-based products like vegetables and mushrooms will provide the added benefit of high-volume foods to bulk up your meals and some extra vitamins and minerals, ensuring you feel great.

These plant-based high protein sources will give you 4-6g of protein per 200g serving, using a significantly small portion of your overall calorie intake.

- Broccoli

- Mushrooms

- Corn

- Spinach

- Kale

- Brussels sprouts

- Artichoke

- Cauliflower

- Beet greens

- Green beans

- Potatoes

- Arugula

- Asparagus

Protein can also be found in dairy products like milk, cheese, and yogurt, like vegetables; dairy products contain important micronutrients like calcium, vitamin D, potassium, magnesium, and vitamin B12. Some dairy products like natural yogurt are also high in probiotics supporting gut health which is important as many diseases start in the gut.

Now let's move on to the next most important macronutrient- fats

Much like carbs, fats have been unfairly put in the "no good" basket regarding macros and weight loss. People are either in the no carbs or no fat camp when we should all be having both. Evolutionarily, humans have always been meant to eat high-fat foods.

Fats give us the most calories per gram, 9 calories compared to 4 from protein and carbs. That worked well back in the caveman era as we were hunter-gatherers and never knew when our next meal would come.

Nowadays, fat is still important, but we do have to be a little careful with how much fat we consume, as those extra calories per gram can add up quickly if you're mindlessly eating. Fats not only taste great, but in many cases, they are hidden; things like butter and oils are often used for cooking foods, and even though you can't see them when your plate is served up, those calories are still there and still count towards your daily intake. Other things like spreads, dressings, and dips that, although they taste great, can also be full of fat and add a lot of extra calories to your meal without adding much volume to bulk up your plate to help keep you full. Things like guacamole, mayonnaise, and Caesar dressing are a few common examples.

Keeping that in mind, we don't want to completely take out all fats from our diet, as Just as proteins and carbs, fats play an important role in our ability to remain in optimal health. Unlike carbs, which you can technically live without and be fine, fats, on the other hand, cannot be eliminated; you cannot live without fat in your diet, or at least you will be very sick if you do.

Here are a few things fat does in your body:

- Fats insulate your body, protecting your vital organs and helping with brain functionality; this is why that last little bit of fat around your stomach is always so hard to get rid of; it's there to protect you.

- Fats help with transportation and absorption of vitamins A, D, E, and K.

- The omega-3 fatty acids EPA and DHA support cardiovascular health, joint health, and digestion.

- Fats slow down the digestion of your food which helps keep you fuller for longer.

- Fats help with balancing your hormones and regulating your mood

Like both of the other macronutrients, there are good and bad fats, monounsaturated and polyunsaturated, along with some good, saturated fats in moderation will keep you in good condition, helping you fight off cardiovascular disease.

Some good sources of fats are the following

- Ghee

- Seeds

- Avocado

- Dark chocolate/cacao nibs

- Olives

- Fatty fish (salmon, mackerel)

- Egg yolks (they get a bad rap sometimes, but in my opinion, they are nature multivitamins)

- Oils (olive, macadamia, and avocado are great, and coconut and MCT oil should also be included in your diet in moderation)

- Nuts

- Pasture-Raised Meat (beef, lamb)

Trans fats, on the other hand, are the bad ones. They are man-made fats that are used mainly because it's cheap and increases a product's shelf life; let's face it, they taste pretty good too. Some bad sources of fats to limit are things like Vegetable oils that are manufactured and hidden in things like crackers, crispy biscuits, microwave pizza, and popcorn.

A general rule of thumb is that you want to make sure 25%-35% of your total calories come from fat.

Now, the last of the macronutrients : Carbohydrates

Before I get into carbs and how they work in your body, I'll start by saying that carbohydrates are the only macro you don't need to survive. You can still maintain a long healthy, and active life without carbs; this is why the keto diet is so popular and successful. However, you have to ask yourself, can you sustain that lifestyle long-term? Can you give up pasta, bread, potatoes, and fruit long-term? If the answer is yes, then a diet like keto might be a great option for you, there are many benefits to it; in fact, I wrote a book about it and tried keto myself for a few months to see what the results would be like and how it made me feel. Although I felt good and lost a stack of weight, I knew full well, being part Italian and my love of pasta, that there was no way I could keep it up. The best diet is the one you can stick to forever, making it a lifestyle, and for that reason, I believe keeping carbs in my diet was the best path forward for me. Carbohydrates are your body's preferred source of energy. Once consumed, carbs get stored in your muscles as glycogen. Over the years, carbs have gotten a bad reputation as the reason for people putting on weight and finding it hard to lose. This is completely false; they are absolutely fine, and eating healthy carbs in the right proportion will keep your muscles and brain strong, healthy, and performing at their best.

Not all carbs are created equal, there are fast-digestion unhealthy carbohydrates like candy bars and ice cream, and then you have your slow-digestion carbohydrates like rice. These are all listed on the glycemic index, which I won't go into here, but you can google if you're interested. In most cases, it's the slow-digestion carbs you want to include in your diet; these are the ones that will give you sustained energy over a longer period rather than that quick sugar hit followed shortly after that by that crash we have all experienced from a late afternoon snack.

When you exercise, carbs are the macronutrient that is most readily available for your body to use as it's the easiest to break down. They also replenish your glycogen stores post-workout and are vital for muscle recovery, good sleep, and overall mood.

Pro-tip, consuming carbohydrates directly after your workout is the one time, I recommend some of those sugary, quicker, releasing carbs as they replenish those glycogen levels faster. Getting those carbs in, along with some quality protein which I will go through in the supplements section, is imperative to your recovery, so if you enjoy a Mars bar, this would be the best time to have one.

Here are a few sources of carbohydrates for you:

- Rice

- Bread

- Pasta

- Oats

- White potato

- Sweet potato

- Greens

- Brussels sprouts

- Broccoli

- Cauliflower

- Onion

- Squash

- Carrots

- Sweet peppers

A Word on Fiber

Dietary fiber is a complex form of carbohydrate, and there are two types, soluble and insoluble, and they both play different roles in the body.

Soluble fiber is soluble in water and helps slow digestion and absorption of food, particularly carbohydrates. This helps regulate blood sugar levels and keep your energy levels from crashing. Soluble fiber is great for your heart, helping lower blood cholesterol levels. It also helps keep you full, which is great when you're eating at a caloric deficit to lose weight.

Some good sources of soluble fiber are

- Oatmeal

- Barley

- Beans

- Nuts

- Apples

- Blueberries

Insoluble fiber, on the other hand, does not combine with water; it helps maintain a healthy digestive system by building up stool volume and speeding up the digestion of food. Vegetables are your best bet to increase insoluble fiber and whole grains.

High fiber foods are full of vitamins and minerals, both soluble and insoluble play a key role in gut health, disease prevention, and weight maintenance, so ensuring you get a good balance of both shouldn't be overlooked. A general guideline for fiber intake is around 10-15 grams per 1000 calories.

Some good high-fiber foods to include in your diet are:

- Apples

- Prunes

- Lentils

- Sweet potatoes

- Beans

- Avocado

- Broccoli

- Raspberries

- Sprouts

- Blackberries

- Asparagus

- Carrots

- Pears

- Corn

- Whole grains

- Oats

- Peas

- Breads

- Pumpkin seeds

- High fiber cereals

Counting calories

I will say that from my experience calorie counting will guarantee success if you get it right and follow the plan. That's a big "IF" though as there is a learning curve at the start where mistakes will be made so it might take a few weeks to get it down properly.

Once you get a handle on it though it takes all of the guesswork out of it. I think it gives you a good understanding of where your calories are coming from and how much you consume daily as most people mindlessly consume way more calories than they think they are and then wonder why they are not losing weight. I still weigh most of my foods to this day, I don't find it takes anymore effort and I enjoy the discipline of it, obviously I don't get too obsessed, if there are foods I can't weigh and record I don't lose sleep over it, I just do the best I can.

I recommend calorie counting for at least the first 4-6 weeks. After that most people would have eaten most of the foods that normally make up their diet so you will get a good idea of the portion sizes you need to be eating and the rough calorie count. At this point you should be well placed to "eyeball" what you put on your plate rather than weighing your meals out all the time.

From there it's just about making small changes, as you get through the 90 days, you will hit plateaus along the way as you lose weight and require less calories. This makes sense as you will be a smaller person carrying less weight and not need as many calories. Don't go overboard with this though, people often go much lower than they need to mess up their hormones and make it impossible to stick with.

Below is a table showing you how to calculate your daily maintenance caloric intake, this means the amount you need to eat just to maintain your current weight. There are many different formulas for calculating calories and macros out there and none are 100% accurate including this one, we are all different and our bodies will react differently to certain amounts calories so this is just a starting point, changes will be made during that learning phase I spoke about earlier depending on how your body reacts and how you are feeling.

Note, for activity level, the majority of people will fit into the middle category of average activity level.

Activity Level

Below Average	Minimal exercise + normal daily activities.
	Bodyweight (lbs.) x 12 calories
Average	1 hour of exercise + normal daily activities 4-5 times per week
	Bodyweight (lbs.) x 14
Above Average	2-3 hours of exercise + normal daily activities 4-5 times per week
	Bodyweight (lbs.) x 16

Once you have calculated your maintenance caloric intake, you must choose a number of calories to take off, putting your body into a caloric deficit to lose weight. When choosing your deficit, you will need to take some things into account. There are pros and cons to different deficit amounts, and each will require a different lifestyle change, so you need to be honest with yourself when choosing which way to go.

The problem I often see here is people choosing to go too aggressive with their calorie deficit; it destroys their confidence when they can't keep it up and leads to them quitting. Don't let this happen to you. Remember, you're not married to your chosen calorie deficit, so if you get this wrong and find it too hard to sustain daily, you can always change it as you go. Like anything, this is a trial and error process; keep making adjustments until you get the plan that suits you and gets results.

The only certainty here is that if you quit, you WILL NOT change your body, so be honest, pick a deficit that you think will allow you to maintain as much of a "normal" lifestyle as you can, and get started.

Understand that the right deficit for you might not be the one that will get you losing weight the fastest, but this is a long-term game.

Here are the different caloric deficits amounts I normally recommend, as well as the pros and cons of each.

Small Deficit

Taking 10-15% of your maintenance calories off daily.

Pro

- This can be accomplished with a very small amount of change to your lifestyle regarding how much food you're eating.

- It will not hinder athletic performance as much since you're eating close to maintenance, so you should have plenty of energy.

Con

- Weight loss is slower due to the deficit being small.

- It's better for people that are already relatively lean.

- You need to be 100% confident in your ability to track food, as there is no margin for error. Even the slightest mistake in tracking can put you back at maintenance or even at a caloric surplus.

Moderate Deficit (recommended for most)

Taking 20-25% of your maintenance calories off daily.

Pro

- Faster fat loss on average

- Can use exercise as well as food restriction to achieve the deficit

- Does not require massive food restriction or increases in activity to achieve

- It allows you to maintain some type of deficit even if you make a mistake here and there with your food tracking.

Con

- It will feel more restricted than the small deficit

- The body will fight back to an extent at first with changes to metabolism and hormones.

Large Deficit

Taking 25% or more of your maintenance calories off daily

Pro

- Maximal fat loss

- You won't have to "diet" for as long since the higher deficit will mean you should reach your result a bit quicker.

- If you're under a time constraint such as needing to be in shape for a not far away wedding, this can be a good way to drop weight fast.

- Difficult to offset the deficit completely with errors in tracking

Con

- With very little food flexibility, you will feel restricted

- The total time people can stick to this is low due to the impact on lifestyle

- Food options become limited as many foods with high-calorie counts will have to be removed altogether.

- It will have the largest impact on your hormone balance and metabolism.

- It can negatively impact your energy for training and everyday life.

Here is an example of how to put this all together and calculate your calories for a female who weighs 170lb with an average activity level and a moderate deficit.

- 170 x 14 = 2380 calories (maintenance level)

- 25% of 2380 = 595 calories (moderate deficit)

- 2380 - 595 = 1785 calories per day is your goal

Macro Calculations

Protein

- 0.8- 1.3G of protein per pound of bodyweight

- 0.82 x 170lb = 139.4 (round up to 140g per day)

- This equals 560 calories (140g x 4 Calories in each gram

Fat 25%-35% of total caloric intake

- 1785 calories per day x 30% = 535.5 round up to 536 calories to be taken in from fats

- 535 calories divided by 9 (9 calories in a gram of fat) = 59.5g of fat round up to 60g

Carbohydrates – whatever calories are left will be in the form of carbs

- 1785 calories per day

- Minus 536 calories coming from fats = 1249 calories

- Minus 560 calories from protein = 689 calories left to come from carbs

- 689 calories divide by 4 (4 calories per gram of carbohydrate)

- Equals 172.25g of carbs per day (round down to 172g)

Final macro breakdown

- 140g protein

- 60g fat

- 172g carbs

The rounding up and down of numbers will mean you change your total daily caloric intake slightly, but that's fine. It's too little to make a difference.

Note: If you want to simplify this further, you don't necessarily have to track all 3 nutrients perfectly. The most important ones to focus on are your overall calorie intake and protein. Aim to get as close as possible to tour calculations for both. As far as fat and carb go, they aren't as important to track, so long as you get a good balance of both, you should be right.

As I said earlier, I think it's a good idea to give this a go, but I know a percentage of you already know they just won't stick to counting calories even for a day. There is an alternative for you guys, but it's not as specific to your individual caloric and macro needs as tracking is. You will have to pay attention to how you feel along the way as this method could easily lead to you under-eating. If your energy or mood drops or you are constantly hungry, adjust slightly with more calories.

I want you to focus on how you set out your plate rather than the calorie content of the foods on it.

See the picture below.

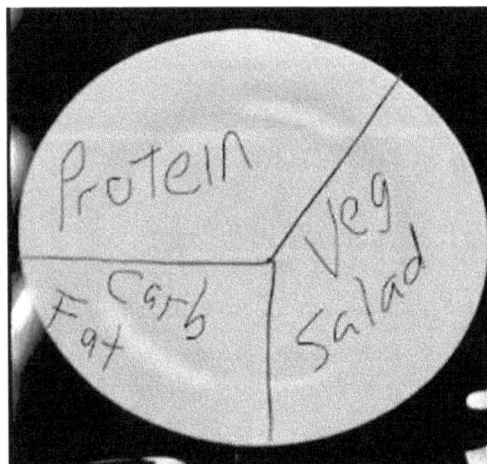

Here we have a balanced meal setup; if you can set out 3 meals a day like this and then add 2 high-protein snacks, such as some Greek yogurt with some blueberries, you should be in pretty good shape to lose weight.

Take up most of your plate with a vegetable/salad and a protein source. The protein option includes beef, steak, chicken breast, eggs, salmon, white fish, tofu, etc.

Once you have your veggies and protein taken care of, the remainder of the plate will come in carbohydrates and healthy fats. You will find that most of your protein sources, except for things like chicken breast or turkey, will also double up as a healthy fat source, so most of the time, you can use the remainder of the plate for carbs.

If you have a lean protein source that doesn't have much fat, adding olive oil or avocado to your salad will allow you to get your fat content in.

Quick pro tip: Do not drink your calories. Since you will be eating at a calorie deficit, you want to be very selective about where those calories come from. On top of being extremely unhealthy, things like sodas and juices have high amounts of calories. The more calories you consume in liquid form, the less you have to play with in the form of solid foods, and it's the solid foods that will satisfy you, making your diet easier to stick to.

Once you get your calories in place, the next thing is to make sure you are getting enough water each day.

Anywhere from 2-3L per day is what I recommend. Not only will water help keep you full in between meals, but it helps keep your skin looking good; it helps to keep your joints cushioned, protects your spinal cord, helps eliminate toxins from your body, helps prevent kidney stones, and maintains an all-around healthier heart.

While we are on the topic of liquids, I want to explore alcohol and how it affects your weight loss.

There is a myth that alcohol makes you fat just because it is alcohol. Yes, if you drink too much alcohol, it will lead to weight gain, but there is more to it than just the extra calories being consumed.

Alcohol is a poison to the body and not something your body wants. Because of this, when you drink it, your body prioritizes getting rid of it as soon as possible. It does this by putting your whole digestive system on hold, slowing down the rate at which food moves through the digestive tract. To try and eliminate it from the body as quickly as possible, it will begin to metabolize the alcohol first in place of any other nutrients in your body, so whatever foods you eat, be it healthy or unhealthy, end up getting stored as fast. In contrast, the body aims to metabolize alcohol first.

On average, it takes around an hour to metabolize a standard drink, so you have a big night out with a lot of drinking. Well, il let you do the math on that one.

Add to this the fact that when we drink, it normally leads to us eating more greasy, high-fat foods that more than likely put us into a calorie surplus compounding its effects.

Am I saying to stop drinking alcohol? No, of course not; I still enjoy a beer or a glass of wine; we are all human, and you must live your life too. Everything is in moderation. It's just something to keep in mind. It will also depend on how fast you want to transform your body. If you have a certain date coming up that you need to achieve by then, you might need to hold yourself more accountable than someone happy just making small gradual improvements over a longer period.

Reading Nutrition Labels

Counting your macros starts with knowing what is in your food; to do this, you need to be able to read and understand nutrition labels.

You will find the nutrition label for most foods on the packaging. Although they can look slightly different depending on the product, brand, and location, they all pretty much have the same information:

Total Fat, Total Carbohydrates, which include dietary fiber and Protein.

Here are the essential things to look at when tracking:

- **SERVING SIZE**: You'll notice that the serving size is given as a cup measurement and as weight. I recommend measuring by weight as cup size differs from country to country.

- **TOTAL FAT**: This includes all fat types (saturated, unsaturated, and trans fats, all 3 should be listed), but it is the total number at the top you should track.

- **TOTAL CARBOHYDRATE**: This includes sugars, which are usually listed separately but use the total carbohydrate number

- **DIETARY FIBER:** You can track fiber using these labels. If it's not listed on the label, the food has no fiber. Fiber doesn't necessarily need to be tracked if weight loss is your only goal, but I'm tipping you probably want to be healthy too, so it's good to make sure you are getting the appropriate amount,

- **PROTEIN:** There will only be one number under protein, so tracking this one is easy.

Tracking Tools

Most people will use an app to track their macros, which makes it super simple now as you can simply scan the barcode or manually type in the food item and the company that makes it and then save it for easier access the next time you eat the same food.

My personal choice is MyFitnessPal, but there are many out there, so find the one that you find most user-friendly.

Supplement guide

Supplements get mixed reactions in the health and fitness world; some people place too much importance on them, while others claim they are just expensive urine.

I stand somewhere in the middle; plenty of overpriced, over-marketed supplements on the market promise the world and deliver an atlas. But at the same time, many should be considered for optimal health.

Things like fat burners, you can stay away from; they may add that .5 of a percent to improving your physique, but that's only if everything else with your diet is perfect.

The meal replacement shakes and companies out there are the other things I would steer away from. There is one major player in this department; while I can't name that company, I'm sure you can probably figure out who they are. They tell you to skip two meals daily and replace them with shakes. This, like any other meal replacement shake system, is a short-term fix that will lure you in with some quick results but let me tell you, unless you are willing to stay on those overpriced shakes for the rest of your life, then at some point you are going to have to come off them. Any weight lost will come back on just as quickly as it dropped off.

You have to learn to lose weight with real food, fitting in the foods you love if you want this to be a sustainable lifestyle that you can do forever because that's what we are looking for here, something we can do forever.

I highly recommend the following supplements, but as with anything else, supplements are not all created equal. There are good and poor brands, and since nutritional supplements in some countries are not regulated and don't have to list everything in them, separating the good from the poor quality can be hard. Always do your research and speak to your doctor before beginning any supplement.

Fish oil

Fish oil supplements give the body essential omega-3 fatty acids, which help regulate inflammation. Omega-3 fatty acids are important to our health, but the body cannot produce them independently; they can only be taken in through food and supplements. An adequate omega-3 has been shown to help maintain a healthy body weight, regulate immune function, and promote muscle and joint health. 500-900mg of omega-3 daily is generally the required amount for most people. Foods like salmon, anchovies, and mackerel are good sources to include in your diet, but supplementing with a good quality fish oil tablet can help you reach the required level.

Protein Powder

This is probably the most common supplement used by people training for strength. I use them and have done so for years. Are they a necessity? No, if you can get enough from food alone, you don't need to supplement it, but most people do not get anywhere near enough protein throughout the day. You need even more than the average couch potato if you are doing resistance training. Even someone like me, who eats protein with every meal, and consumes plenty of turkey, eggs, and chicken, struggles to reach the amount needed. Protein makes you feel full, and you don't need much of it before it becomes a struggle to finish; this is where supplements can be beneficial and convenient. Just ensure you don't go overboard with them; most of your protein needs to be coming in through food intake, not supplementation.

In all cases, the quality of your protein will be much better through food, there is only one time where I would say a supplement is optimal over food, and that's post-workout. After your workout, your body is depleted and needs protein and carbs as soon as possible. This is where a supplement can be a better option as it digests quicker and gets into your system a lot sooner than solid food that has to be chewed, swallowed, and digested, and that takes time. Below is a brand I use and highly rate; it's an Australian company that sells quality grass-fed protein. They ship worldwide; if you are interested, click the link and have a look, but once again, do your research before using.

Blackbelt Protein and Supplements

Creatine

You may or may not have heard of creatine, and if you have, you probably have the idea in your head that it's a bodybuilding supplement only used by men and other meatheads at the gym, but I can assure you creatine is just as important for women. It is the most researched supplement on the market and the safest. Creatine is an amino acid stored in our muscles and brain as an energy source. When we need energy, our bodies convert creatine into phosphocreatine, which fuels our muscles. Creatine has been shown to help women, in particular, add lean muscle, helping sustain high energy levels and mental clarity throughout a workout; Creatine is found in most meat sources like liver, kidneys, red meat, pork, and fish but like protein, most people do not get enough from diet alone. If you're vegan or vegetarian, you would benefit greatly from adding a creatine supplement into your daily routine. This is one supplement I recommend everyone take.

Greens powder

While this one isn't necessary, we can all agree that we probably don't take in anywhere near the amount of vegetables we should be each day. If you are one of the few that do, then there is no need for a greens powder, but if you're like me, then they are a handy way to supplement your veggie intake, but in no way should they replace eating broccoli, kale, and spinach. A good greens powder contains high levels of vitamins and minerals associated with maintaining a healthy immune system. They have Vitamin A anti-inflammatory properties that enhance immunity; Selenium is a good example. It is found in most greens powders, proven to help the immune system fight infection. This is one of those supplements that don't taste all that great, and to be honest, if you find one that does, then it's probably not the healthiest one to take.

Multi vitamin

A good quality multivitamin is probably one of the most important supplements you can include in your diet. No matter how much you watch what you eat, it's pretty hard to ensure you're getting all the micronutrients you require to run at optimal health. Not only are most people not getting in their standard recommended fruit and vegetable intake daily, but there have also been studies showing that due to things like the depletion and quality of soil these days, food today contains fewer vitamins and minerals than 20-plus years ago. Taking a multivitamin on top of a nutritious diet will ensure you top up on everything you need to.

Probiotic

Probiotics are important for gut health, making them an important addition to your supplement plan. The gut has good and bad bacteria in it, the bad bacteria is what normally causes many diseases and illness, what a good probiotic does is help balance that out by giving you some good bacteria. Probiotics help regulate inflammation, immune function, brain health and weight management. An imbalance between the bad and good bacteria in your gut can also lead to nutrient deficiencies even if you have a good diet and are supplementing.

Sleep

One of the most overlooked parts of transforming your body physically is getting a good amount of quality sleep each night; Sleep is when our muscles repair themselves, grow, and get stronger.

World champion cross-fitter Matt Fraser said in an interview that if sleep wasn't normal, it would be a bad substance; that's how big of an effect it has on your performance.

Most people need 7-8 hours of sleep each night; I know this is something we don't always have control over. I can tell you from personal experience that I struggle in this department. My brain always wants to kick into overdrive when my head hits the pillow worrying about anything and everything.

Getting less than 7 hours of sleep a night does have a negative effect on weight loss; one thing that insufficient sleep leads to is binge eating. I have been in that situation many times where I have been tired and hit the cupboard opting for junk foods, maybe to make myself feel better.

A lack of sleep will mess with your metabolism as it triggers a cortisol spike, cortisol for those that don't know is the stress hormone; in this instance, it will tell your body to conserve energy to fuel your following day as it knows the lack of sleep from the previous night is going to mean energy levels are depleted. In simple terms, you will hang onto current body fat stores.

It also hampers your body's ability to process insulin, the hormone that helps change food into energy. When this happens, your body doesn't process the fat from your bloodstream properly, resulting in it being stored as fat.

It can also bring on things like high blood pressure, poor cognitive performance, memory consolidation, premature aging, and negatively affect overall mood.

Yes, sleep is hard to get sometimes with many things out of your control but try your hardest to get a good amount each night by setting up a nighttime routine and being disciplined.

Chapter 7:

Work on Your Inside Game

The following chapter will discuss what it means to think and live like a champion and how the examples of high achievers can serve you in your commitment to losing weight and attaining optimal health. It will also address behavioral eating, the all too common tendency to understate the dangers of self-sabotaging habits, and how a refusal to accept responsibility can make progress impossible. Pursuing weight loss and transforming your body can be discouraging in a modern society that shames and, at the same time, enables unhealthy eating habits, and it is important to keep a positive outlook. This chapter will explore the basic psychology behind losing weight and the benefits of self-affirmation, self-acceptance, and the setting of tangible goals.

Also discussed will be the principle of maintaining optimism when surrounded by a negative environment and people around you., as well as several strategies for protecting yourself against criticism that isn't constructive and moving your objectives steadily. Challenging and rewarding yourself appropriately will depend, above all, on your mentality and the effort you put into your diet and exercise regimen. In that spirit, the chapter will conclude with several ideas for instilling a winning mindset into your commitment to losing weight and other areas of your everyday life.

What makes a champion? Whether you are an aspiring Olympic gold medalist or simply someone struggling, as so many of us do, to honor their commitments to their health and well-being, it is important to realize that without desire, it will be very difficult, if not impossible, to succeed in your goals. A true desire for the reward of optimal health is the remedy to a fear of the consequences of failure or inactivity, and it is the best motive to succeed. Fear of failure is paralytic, whereas elite athletes often describe the desire for success to be their primary driving force and that which gives them the energy to push past pain and fatigue. Muhammad Ali once said, "I hated every minute of training, but I said, 'Don't quit. Suffer now and live the rest of your life as a champion.'" Seeing today's challenges as tomorrow's achievements is vital to understanding the thought process of those who dare to set lofty goals and the perseverance to accomplish them.

Failure, at some time, in some respect, is inevitable in the pursuit of any highly demanding goal, and it is in this defining moment of the process that everybody faces a choice: allow failure to define their self-image or allow it to serve as a valuable lesson, and reinforce their commitment to self-improvement. Champions do not make excuses for their shortcomings, nor do they judge themselves or attempt to place blame on others. They simply take stock of the factors that led to their failure and return to the task with a newfound understanding of what it will take to bypass the roadblocks to success. Even Michael Jordan, who is by most accounts the greatest basketball player of all time, has experienced failure. "I've missed more than 9,000 shots in my career." He states. "I've lost almost 300 games, 26 times. I've been trusted to take the game-winning shot and missed. I've failed over and over and over again in my life, and that is why I succeed.

Winning, as it applies to direct competition and in life, is the product of high expectations of yourself, a sense of due diligence in preparation, and a presence of mind in execution. It is not something that happens as the result of luck or circumstance but by the investment of effort greater than the sum of the obstacles to victory. It happens only when you fully understand that there is no way around the hard work necessary to defeat whatever is in your path and that all success will depend on your efforts. Unlike those who give up at the first sign of hardship or defeat themselves with vague, unreachable goals, winners set goals that are, at once, specific to their obstacles, measurable in terms of improvement, realistic to their abilities, and on a time-specific deadline. They are humble enough to consider their limitations when forming a plan. Yet, they take themselves seriously enough to expect great results, planning to make their desires a reality and then applying all possible effort in completing the action.

By this definition, "winners" and "losers" are not determined by the outcome of a competition but by the quality of their efforts. Being a winner means seeing yourself as someone who can accomplish great things and knowing that you have genuinely done everything in your power to reach your objectives. It means not shying away from challenges, being deterred by failures, or coming up with reasons to quit. It means striving, regardless of circumstance and natural ability, to improve and honor your commitments and well-being by showing up, one day at a time. The only way to "lose," in the larger sense, is to give up on yourself or decide that you aren't even going to try. The fact that you have chosen to lose weight and get strong through dieting and exercise means that you are already a winner; now, it is only a matter of discovering your greatest potential and setting out to make your desire a reality.

No matter how tough, no matter what kind of outside pressure, no matter how many bad breaks along the way, I must keep my sights on the final goal, to win, win, win- and with more love and passion than the world has ever witnessed in any performance. -
Billie Jean King

The Hard Truth

The ability to identify obstacles to success will depend greatly on learning to understand what constitutes an obstacle and how to plan realistically to overcome it. In many cases, the most daunting roadblocks to losing weight are related to psychological factors, like unconscious behavioral eating or resistance to hard work, which can make identifying them a difficult and humbling experience. Self-awareness is a quality that comes not only from acknowledging our strengths but examining our weaknesses, and we only do ourselves a disservice when we distort the truth in our minds or pretend that a problem doesn't exist. Learning about the numerous medical concerns associated with being overweight can prove ample motivation for some to begin pursuing better health, but those who ignore the reality often consign themselves to defeat from the outset. When it comes to being truthful, you don't have to tell anybody anything you don't want to, as long as you don't lie to yourself.

As we see from the mentality of those who achieve at high levels, "winning" is simply giving ourselves a chance to win, and "losing" is nothing more than making the decision not to try. A lack of motivation can ensure a lack of progress and must be addressed, like any other roadblock, if it is to be conquered. It will not help to spend time making excuses for it, blaming others, or waiting for the perfect set of circumstances to provide a means of overcoming it.

One of my favorite quotes is by the late Greg Pitt; it's a quote that I can relate to "Life isn't about waiting for the storm to pass; it's about learning how to dance in the rain."

Only by accepting personal responsibility for lack of effort will it be possible to discover the incentives to get you out of bed and working out and keep you focused and committed to your efforts. Later chapters will present strategies for finding personal motivation to work out consistently.

The truth is that no matter how you dress up, the challenge of staying on your diet and exercise regimen and losing weight is real, and there will not be any shortcuts or ways to get around doing the necessary amount of work. To lose a pound of fat, you will have to burn 3,500 more calories than you consume, which means that your plan will have to be structured with the correct balance of strength training and cardio to complement that. This is the only way to lead to significant weight loss when combined with healthier eating habits and enough sleep. Diet pills, especially the over-the-counter variety, often have little to no effect and can even lead to serious health concerns. Of the four approved prescription weight loss medications, all have side effects, and some carry the risk of seizures and death. The reward of losing weight is not remotely worth the risk involved with taking a largely untested, possibly fatal substance, and this option should not be considered a viable alternative to healthy, natural methods. To achieve your ideal body, you must cultivate a positive outlook and embrace the more demanding aspects of the journey. Learn to enjoy the journey and the small victories along the way, and leave the counters bullshit to those looking for a quick fix that will ultimately fail.

Weight Loss is 80% Psychology

Mind over matter, as with training for an athletic competition, losing weight depends not only on a program of diet and exercise to achieve it but also on a strong, focused mind to stay on course, and the endeavor can often require a similar level of devotion and psychological resilience. It is a competition against outside forces, such as the difficulty in finding healthy food options in the modern world where it seems there is a McDonald's or a Wendy's on every corner, as well as a much greater struggle against internal obstacles; fear, complacency, embarrassment, doubt, self-pity, addiction, etc., and winning in this competition means maintaining focus and a positive mindset. Unfortunately, people trying to lose weight are continually given the message by the dieting and fitness industries, often as well as those around them, that somehow, there is something morally wrong with them and that they should be ashamed for even being in such a position. Reacting to this notion of "shame" put forward by others is allowing yourself to be motivated by a need for their acceptance, and as a result, you can become less self-motivated and self-accepting. Many who experience this issue have found that shame can easily lead to anger, and anger can lead to eventual rebellion against their diet and exercise programs. While being self-motivated is a more complex task than being motivated by others, it is ultimately more positive, fulfilling, and likely to succeed in the long run.

Becoming healthy is, in many ways, its reward, but by the same token, being unhealthy can lead to depression, anxiety, and a distorted viewpoint on health in general. It can be difficult in such cases to be motivated by the prospect of feeling healthy, as the feeling is unfamiliar, and the rewards can sometimes appear distant. A sense of feeling better can only come from starting the process and discovering the benefits of consistent, healthy choices. The knowledge that you are taking and are continuing to take steps towards improving longevity and your quality of life can greatly diminish stress and is, for many, the greatest motivating factor behind the commitment to lose weight. The nature of a goal like losing a large amount of weight is that it can take a long time to see encouraging progress in terms of pounds lost. Some have found it helpful to set more short-term goals, such as counting calories, energy levels, the natural high you get after you finish a workout, improving body mass index, blood pressure, and cholesterol, or simply taking a sense of achievement from milestones relating to diet and exercise (days spent dieting, miles run, personal bests for pushups, etc.). Whatever the motive is for getting in shape, it is important that it is your own and not someone else's and that it is a positive force in your life, capable of helping you push through the difficult days and make the most of the easier ones. Remember that any step towards doing right by yourself, even a small one, is a step in the right direction, and you should be proud of yourself for every effort you make.

Falling in Love with the Process

There are few rewards more desirable than having an ideal body and the confidence that comes with those transfers into other areas of your life. But as a champion knows, a reward is the culmination of a process, and without investing the required time and energy, that process cannot be completed. Losing weight is a game of increments and steady progress, and the more you can learn to love the entire experience of diet and exercise, the easier it will be to get into a consistent routine. A positive outlook on each separate element of the program can help identify which of them you might find enjoyable and even become the reason you work out when you feel tired or persevere in your diet when obstacles show themselves along the way. It can also be useful to add other elements that make the routine more enjoyable without taking anything from its effectiveness.

A common practice among people beginning a fitness regimen is to convince a friend to join them in the activity or find a like-minded connection with someone they can compare notes. Having a workout buddy can give perspective regarding your efforts, and having someone to encourage you when you want to give up can make all the difference. Additionally, having someone else involved means you will be more likely to make and keep appointments to work out because even though you might be able to justify letting yourself down, you sure won't want to let your friend down. These factors, amongst others, are said to account for the increased levels of reported weight loss among people who exercise with friends.

For some, the feeling alone of sweating out toxins, strengthening the heart, and shedding pounds is ample reason to love the exercise process. They see the activity as a relief from stress rather than as a cause of it, and they find it motivating to record their improvements and push for new personal bests. Another way to add incentive is to engage regularly in sports and recreational physical activities, which is also an excellent way to stay in shape; basketball, swimming, and soccer can be a far more enjoyable form of cardio than riding a stationary bike for 40 minutes as long as the activity is treated as a serious method of exercise with goals, time-based commitments, and a sense of the larger picture.

Other personality types find the prospect of physical exertion tedious and have more success staying focused when an outside distraction, such as music, is added to the mix. Being distracted by music or even a podcast can take the mind away from the more discomforting factors of a hard workout and can have a positive and enhancing influence on energy and outlook.

Smash Your Behavioural Eating

Like most addictions, food addiction is largely triggered by negative thoughts and habits and is widely considered to be primarily psychological. Unlike a habit involving a harmful substance, however, this only becomes detrimental when it is out of balance. That being said, food filled with addictive substances like sodium and high fructose corn syrup is becoming increasingly difficult to avoid, even when actively attempting to do so, and breaking the cycle of a bad habit can often require innovative solutions. Like the champion athlete, who understands that there is no way around hard work, anybody attempting to curb their caloric intake must also understand that there is no other way around their obstacles than to eat healthier and less. Everybody has a different biological makeup and thought process, which means that finding what works for you is a matter of trying different approaches and choosing one that makes sense and feels right. The right weight loss plan is the one that is sustainable; if that's the Keto diet, then go for it; if that's the paleo diet, that's all good as well; if it's flexible dieting that you are able to stick to long term, then that is the right choice for you.

One strategy that has been effective in certain cases is to lay out your diet in such a way that breakfast is the most substantial meal of the day and dinner is the least. A large breakfast, followed by a smaller lunch and an even smaller dinner, is a sequence shown in studies to lead to less hunger throughout the day and a reduced likelihood of cravings leading to unconscious snacking. As the saying goes, "Eat breakfast like a king, lunch like a prince, and dinner like a pauper." If this does not seem to prevent later meals from becoming equally rich, then the intermittent fasting approach mentioned earlier could be the way to get past this, eliminating breakfast and having only lunch, dinner, and a light snack or dessert within a predetermined window of time (e.g., lunch at 12 pm, dinner at 8 pm, and nothing outside of those hours).

Many other programs and thought processes are being tested, and sticking with any plan will be much easier if it doesn't feel like a burden or a punishment. For many, behavior modification therapy can be necessary, while others find a more direct Spartan regimen to better suit their lifestyles. Again, reducing unconscious eating is all about finding the approach to which you are most likely to stay committed and making a tangible change for the better.

Shut the Negative People Out, They Don't Want You to Succeed

Keeping a positive outlook while dieting can be difficult enough in a vacuum, much less when trying to overcome the harmful and judgmental messages put out by those who either mean well and fail to encourage or do not mean well and succeed in discouraging. Criticism is only constructive when it comes from a place of empathy and caring and when it is carefully considered. Needless to say, most critical remarks do not meet these criteria. Instead, they seem as though they were designed to diminish, sabotage, or transfer negative emotion, and no good can come from internalizing them. It is often very telling whether or not the criticism directed towards you was when you had just accomplished something or discussed the idea of doing something positive with your life. Jealousy and resentment can be carefully disguised and extend beyond obvious factors; people can be resentful simply because you feel happier than they do or even because of a perceived attitude towards them that has no basis in truth. Your success puts a spotlight on their shortcomings, and it is easier to drag others down than it is to elevate yourself, and recognizing this motive in people is a big part of keeping the things they say from influencing your process.

Too often, we play into the hands of negative people, either doing or saying nothing in response, trying to ignore them, attacking back, or even changing our behavior to fit their definitions of how we should be. All of these responses are changes in our normal behavior, which is exactly what the critics want. If you are on a long-term diet or fitness plan, anything other than staying true to your goals will only make things harder, so you should always continue to do exactly what you were doing before, regardless of what other people say. Staying committed to your ideas and practices shows them that they have no effect on you and that their attempts to bring you down to their level only make you stronger and surer of your position. It is impossible to please everyone; making one person happy will make another angry, and vice versa. Not only that but by attempting to please everyone, you will end up walking a path that is not what you had planned and losing all focus relating to your goals. Keep in mind that whatever you do, if you do it right, there will always be somebody with something negative to say about it. The best way to disempower that person is to demonstrate that you stand by your actions and beliefs and that their efforts do not affect yours. Unfortunately, a lot of the time, these comments can come from the people closer to us.

Not all criticism, however, is ill-intended or invalid. Sometimes, an outside perspective can show you something you would not have seen on your own and help you improve. Constructive criticism should be recognized when received and considered carefully before it is given. If it is objective, specific, unassuming, and includes recommendations on improving, it is likely coming from a position of good intent and is more likely to ring true. If the advice could help you in your process, you should have the self-recognition not to reject it simply because it is critical. Having the maturity, clarity, and responsibility to weigh helpful advice for its validity is essential to gaining any benefits and is an essential element of success.

Of all the critics in your life, both constructive and destructive, the one you have to live with every day is yourself. We can all be our worst enemies, largely due to the things we tell ourselves about ourselves. Negative self-talk is something I have had to deal with for years, most of my life, and I continue to work on it to this day as it is my natural default setting. Like a negative message from other people, negative self-talk leads to the same issue of becoming distracted from your goals but is often much more influential. As with outside perspectives relating to you, it is good to determine if the message is potentially helpful and, if not, to continue what you were doing before and more of it. This will prove to others and yourself that only you have the power to determine your thoughts and actions and that you will not be distracted or derailed from anything you put your mind to. Remaining focused on the goal, while easier said than done, is always the best way to overcome an obstacle, especially in the case of harmful ideas. You are pursuing a worthwhile pursuit and have every reason to feel good about yourself and your actions.

Reward Yourself

Recognizing and endorsing your accomplishments now and then is essential when pursuing a long-term goal like weight loss, not only for the added incentive but to acknowledge and celebrate that a certain milestone has been reached. Positive reinforcement in the form of a well-deserved reward increases the likelihood of continued proactive behavior and provides something to look forward to in the more immediate future. This does not mean going back to old habits or blowing your diet right out of the water, but instead, finding a fun, interesting way to celebrate your progress; it may mean buying yourself something you were debating whether or not to spend the money on. Whatever it is and whatever the method might be, rewarding yourself creates a cause-and-effect relationship to your routine and helps you to see all of the smaller achievements you've made on the way to your end goal.

How you reward yourself is less important than why, but the more it feels like a reward, the more likely you are to work for it. Going on a vacation, taking a "vacation day," or simply allowing yourself to relax with a sauna or spa treatment can be the perfect way to escape and unwind after weeks to months of hard work, and it is good for your health at the same time. Incentives relating to the goal help maintain focus and remind us that while we may have accomplished something now, there is still a larger goal to move towards.

If you find giving yourself something unrelated to the process is more helpful, the same principle applies; go on a shopping trip, or buy something online, like non-workout clothes or a new device, to have a reminder of your accomplishments in hand. Getting out of the house and attending a movie, concert, or sporting event is a great way to celebrate your achievements with friends and family. Rewarding yourself is a matter of knowing yourself, and your definition of a "reward" may differ entirely from any of the discussed options - but because the ultimate goal of your hard work will not be gained overnight, it will be important to celebrate smaller milestones along the way.

Chapter 8:

Before You Get Started, How Do You Track Progress?.

First take you before photos

Take you before photos wearing an outfit that clearly shows your current body shape, either your underwear or maybe some activewear (remember these photos are for your eyes only)

Take photos of yourself with the following poses.

- Facing front with your hands by your side, completely relaxed

- Facing the front with your arms up and bent as if to flex your biceps. I want you to tense every muscle you can in this photo, your arms, stomach, and legs.

- Facing sideways, completely relaxed with your arms by your side.

- Facing back to the camera, completely relaxed.

- Facing back with the same tense pose you did for your front.

Don't skip this step; you will want to have these photos on hand to compare progress throughout your journey.

As you get further into the program, you will notice that, at some point, your results slow down on the scale; it's inevitable and happens to everyone. You must realize that this doesn't mean you're no longer make progress

This is where the photos come into play; you will be strength training and, therefore, putting on lean muscle, which means, at some point, that will counteract the fat loss resulting in the number on the scale slowing down even though you continue to lose fat. Photos, measurements, and how your clothes fit will show this.

Aim to take a new set of photos maybe every 4-6 weeks with the same outfit on and poses.

Weigh yourself

Yes, I still want you to weigh yourself; I want you to weigh yourself every day, first thing in the morning, with no clothes on, after you go to the bathroom and before you consume food and drink.

I want you to weigh in every day because there are so many things that make the scale weight fluctuate from day to day. Things like how much you ate the day before, how late you had your last meal, how much you drank, what kind of foods you ate, hormone levels, etc. These things can make the scale go up even though you haven't gained any fat.

When you weigh yourself once a week as many do, you are not getting the whole story of your week but rather just the story of the previous 24 hours, as many of the variables I listed above can impact the result and mess with your head. I have had my weight go up by over 1.5kg overnight before while still eating at a deficit, and there is no way I put in 1.5kg of fat in 24 hours; that's virtually impossible.

I want you to weigh in every day; you will see that your weight probably goes up and down each day, much like the stock market, which is normal; I then want you to record your lowest weight of the week; that's the number to pay attention to each week,

Measurements (every 2 weeks and record)

Take a tape measure out and measure around the following areas every two to three weeks, as with weighing yourself make sure all of the conditions are the same. Do it first thing in the morning, after you have gone to the bathroom and before you eat or drink anything.

Back - measure all the way around your body with the tape measure under your arm pits

Hips – measure around the biggest and widest part of your hips.

Stomach – measure both around your belly button and around the narrowest part of your stomach.

Thighs (both left and right), around the thickest part of your thigh

Arm (both left and right), around the middle of your upper arm, halfway between your shoulder and elbow.

Chapter 9:

Quick Start Guide

To get the most out of this program, make sure you do the following steps

1) Read the program in its entirety and watch the videos by using the clickable links or the QR codes in the exercise descriptions. Most of the questions you're going to have will be answered throughout the book. If anything isn't, you can let me know in the Facebook group.

2) Get organized; before you begin the program, download a free calorie counter app to your phone and familiarize yourself with it. I use MyFitnessPal, but there are many out there, so find one you like; the free versions are all you need. Practice tracking for a couple of days prior to starting. Make sure you have a good food scale that works and is accurate, then work out your schedule of when you're going to work out, do your grocery shopping, and when you are going to meal prep. Remember the 6 P's Poor Planning Prevents Piss Poor Performance. It's so true. Don't underestimate it.

3) Calculate your daily caloric intake and your macro split, specifically your protein intake. If you haven't done that already from the earlier chapter, remember to adjust when needed. Only adjust after you have given a set calorie intake for a good 3 to 4 weeks

Remember the calculations

Activity Level – You will more than likely fit into the Average category but if you find yourself exercising less then maybe try below average.

| Below Average | Minimal exercise + normal daily activities. Bodyweight (lbs.) x 12 calories |
| Average | 1 hour of exercise + normal daily activities 4-5 times per week Bodyweight (lbs.) x 14 |

Choose your deficit, you can go back and recap the pros and cons of each deficit in the earlier chapter to help you make your choice. More often than not the moderate deficit is the way to go To get the most out of this program, make sure you do the following steps

1) Read the program in its entirety and watch the videos by using the clickable links or the QR codes in the exercise descriptions. Most of the questions you're going to have will be answered throughout the book. If anything isn't, you can let me know in the Facebook group.

2) Get organized; before you begin the program, download a free calorie counter app to your phone and familiarize yourself with it. I use MyFitnessPal, but there are many out there, so find one you like; the free versions are all you need. Practice tracking for a couple of days prior to starting. Make sure

you have a good food scale that works and is accurate, then work out your schedule of when you're going to work out, do your grocery shopping, and when you are going to meal prep. Remember the 6 P's Poor Planning Prevents Piss Poor Performance. It's so true. Don't underestimate it.

3) Calculate your daily caloric intake and your macro split, specifically your protein intake. If you haven't done that already from the earlier chapter, remember to adjust when needed. Only adjust after you have given a set calorie intake for a good 3 to 4 weeks.

Small Deficit

Taking 10-15% of your maintenance calories off daily

Moderate Deficit (recommended for most)

Taking 20-25% of your maintenance calories off daily

Large Deficit

Taking 25% or more of your maintenance calories off daily

Here are the same examples I showed in the nutrition chapter for calculating your calories and macros for a lady who weighs 170lb with an average activity level.

To get the most out of this program, make sure you do the following steps

1) Read the program and watch the videos using the clickable links or the QR codes in the exercise descriptions. Most of the questions you will have will be answered throughout the book. You can let me know in the Facebook group if anything isn't.

2) Get organized; before you begin the program, download a free calorie counter app and familiarize yourself. I use MyFitnessPal, but there are many out there, so find one you like; the free versions are all you need. Practice tracking for a couple of days prior to starting. Make sure you have a good food scale that works and is accurate, then work out your schedule of when you're going to work out, do your grocery shopping, and when you are going to meal prep. Remember the 6 P's Poor Planning Prevents Piss Poor Performance. It's so true. Don't underestimate it.

3) Calculate your daily caloric intake and macro split, specifically your protein intake. If you haven't done that already from the earlier chapter, remember to adjust when needed. Only adjust after you have been given a set calorie intake for a good 3 to 4 weeks.

- 170 x 14 = 2380 calories (maintenance level)

- 25% of 2380 = 595 calories

- 2380 - 595 = 1785 calories per day is your goal

Macro split

Macro calculations

Protein

- 0.8- 1.3G of protein per pound of bodyweight

- 0.82 x 170lb = 139.4 (round up to 140g per day)

- This equals 560 calories (140g x 4 Calories in each gram)

Fat 25%-35% of total caloric intake

- 1785 calories per day x 30% = 5

- 35.5 round up to 536 calories to be taken in from fats

- 535 calories divided by 9 (9 calories in a gram of fat) = 59.5g of fat round up to 60g

Carbohydrates – whatever calories are left will be in the form of carbs

- 1785 calories per day

- Minus 536 calories coming from fats = 1249 calories

- Minus 560 calories from protein = 689 calories left to come from carbs

- 689 calories divide by 4 (4 calories per gram of carbohydrate)

- Equals 172.25g of carbs per day (round down to 172g)

Final macro breakdown

- **140g protein**

- **60g fat**

- **172g carbs**

If you're not up for tracking macros, you can use the plate setup method for your meals and see how it goes.

4) Write your goals down and get as specific as you can, really go deep here

- Why are you doing this?

- What is the end goal that you're trying to achieve?

- Why is that end goal so important for you?

- How will reaching that goal change your life for the better?

5) Be present. This is important; when I say be present, it means you live in the moment and accept who you are in all its glory. Understand that you are good enough right now and will just make some improvements along the way. Don't worry about how many times you have failed to achieve your body goals in the past, and don't stress about whether or not you think you can achieve them this time. Be present at the moment and

take it one day at a time. Understand you will make mistakes along the way, and that's ok; we all do; I do all the time. If you have a blowout with your calories or go overboard with a meal, you will pick yourself up and get back on track at your next meal. No rule says you have to wait until the next day or Monday to restart, that just maximizes and adds more damage denting your confidence more than it should.

Chapter 10:

The Routine Structure

Weeks 1-8

To be performed Monday, Wednesday, and Friday or any 3 days that you wish throughout the week, try your best to make sure there is at least 1 day off in between workouts to do your walking or rucking and give your muscles a chance to recover from the previous session, also remember to alternate from week to week. In week one, you will do 2x upper body workouts on Monday and Friday and 1x lower body workout on Wednesday; then in week 2, you will flip that around by doing 2 x lower body workouts and 1x upper body workout.

Over the next 8 weeks, you will work on your progressions in these key movements. Once you reach the prescribed rep range on all 3 sets of a particular exercise, move on to the next progression.

Perform as a slow circuit, doing 1 set of each exercise with 2-3 minutes off between each exercise to recover and repeat for 4 rounds. Remember and stretch after your workout for added recovery.

Upper body

- Pike press progression- 3 sets 8-10

- Black widows-3 sets 15

- Door Jam Row- 3 sets 15

- Push-up progression- 3 sets 15

- Dips progression- 3 sets 15

- Heel taps- 3 sets 15 until failure

Lower body

- Squat progression- 3 sets 15

- Glute and lower back progression- 3 sets 15

- Sumo squat- 3 sets 15

- Sumerians - 3 sets 15

- Step ups- 3 sets, 15 each leg

- Fire hydrant- 3 sets until failure

- Side plank- 2 sets on each side for as long as you can

Week 9-12

Over the next 4 weeks, I want to take the same routine, but this time you will perform them as a Tabata workout.

For those of you unfamiliar with Tabata workouts, they are an interval-style workout where you work for 20 seconds and then have a 10-second break for a total of 8 rounds; this will take 4 minutes to complete and is usually timed to music. I want you to perform 4 Tabata workouts per session, which will take you 16 minutes at 4 minutes per workout; just keep alternating between the exercises throughout the rounds exactly as you have been. You can take 3-5 minutes in between workouts to recover.

The smaller breaks add conditioning to your workouts while staying in the desired rep range. These few weeks will also serve you well by shocking the system. Your body is smart and will always find the most efficient way to do things and stay in its comfort zone as long as possible. When it gets used to doing the same exercises at the same rep range and tempo for a long time, like 8 weeks, then it becomes used to it and isn't forced to adapt to the stress it is being put under much like it would have when you first began the program. This is when you need to switch things up and shock your body with a new stimulus.

Doing the workout in a Tabata format will probably require you to go back to a previous progression you have already mastered since you won't be having 2-minute breaks in between sets to fully recover.

To time yourself during these workouts, you can either just use the stopwatch on your phone or go on YouTube and type in "Tabata music" It will come up with a few options of music already timed specifically for these workouts.

After this 4 week's block, you will have done 12 weeks of solid training. You may not be able to perform the hardest progression on every exercise yet. From here, I would recommend taking a week off and giving your body a rest while continuing your walking and stretching. After this, you will repeat from week one, starting at whichever progression you ended at.

Conclusion

This brings us to the end of the program; first of all, I would like to thank you for choosing this book and putting your faith in me to help you transform your body. I do not doubt that if you stick with it, your body will be noticeably different, both with the number on the scale and your body composition.

I would love to hear about your results in the Facebook group, so post your success there; it will help inspire others at the beginning of their journey. Likewise, if you are struggling, contact me via the Facebook group, and I will help you in any way I can.

It might only be something small that needs to be tweaked to get you on the right track. If you have any problems with any of the exercise progressions, such as an injury preventing you from being able to perform it or simply your strength isn't at the level to do it yet, then reach out, and I can give you an alternative.

Click the link, answer the 3 questions, and I look forward to welcoming you into the group.

Also, don't forget to grab your 28-day habit tracker, 21-Day Fat Loss Kickstart plan, Fix your nutrition eBook, and 30% discount on my 12-week coaching program. Click here, fill out your details, and I will send your discount code and the rest of your freebies to your inbox instantly.

If you have any questions about my coaching program, feel free to shoot me an email at michael.zollo@hotmail.com

References

Paturel, A. (2022, August 14). *Does Sleep Affect Weight Loss?*. WebMD. https://www.webmd.com/diet/sleep-and-weight-loss

Pacheco, D., & Wright, H. (2022, April 14). *Physical Health and Sleep: How are They Connected?*. Sleep Foundation. https://www.sleepfoundation.org/physical-healthhttps://www.sleepfoundation.org/physical-health

Join - Working Against Gravity. (n.d.). Working Against Gravity. https://www.workingagainstgravity.com/join

www.ingramcontent.com/pod-product-compliance
Lightning Source LLC
Chambersburg PA
CBHW080400030426
42334CB00024B/2950